P9-DFF-058

WE HAVE AIDS

We Have AIDS

ELAINE LANDAU

Franklin Watts 1990 New York London Toronto Sydney

133541

Library of Congress Cataloging-in-Publication Data

Landau, Elaine.
We have AIDS / Elaine Landau.
p.   cm.
Includes bibliographical references.
Summary: The personal accounts of nine children with AIDS,
discussing their families' reactions, their search for medical
treatment, and their hopes for an eventual cure.
ISBN 0-531-15152-2—ISBN 0-531-10898-8 (lib. bdg.)
1. AIDS (Disease) in children—Juvenile literature.   [1. AIDS
(Disease)]   I. Title.
RJ387.A25L36   1990
362.1'9892'979200922—dc20   89-24801   CIP   AC

Copyright © 1990 by Elaine Landau
All rights reserved
Printed in the United States of America
6   5   4   3   2   1

Also by Elaine Landau

ALZHEIMER'S DISEASE
LYME DISEASE
THE SIOUX
SURROGATE MOTHERS
TROPICAL RAIN FORESTS AROUND
THE WORLD

For A. J. & K. S., who were
interviewed for this book
and are no longer with us.
Two outstanding young people
who enriched the lives of
all who knew them.

CONTENTS

WE HAVE AIDS

INTRODUCTION

AIDS is a painfully devastating disease. At this time, it is still incurable. AIDS is an equal-opportunity killer, striking anyone, regardless of age, ethnic or religious background, or family income. No matter where you live or what kind of family you're from, if you don't have the facts about AIDS, you are vulnerable to the disease.

No one is magically immune to illness or tragedy. Wishing or thinking that you'll be safe doesn't make it so. A recent survey of Boston, Massachusetts, teenagers between the ages of sixteen and nineteen revealed that 70 percent were sexually active. However, out of the 15 percent who indicated taking precautions to avoid AIDS, only 5 percent used effective measures. To worsen the situation, AIDS has made the ultimate consequences of intravenous drug use even deadlier.

With the onset of the AIDS epidemic, the stakes have become exceedingly high. Once the disease has been contracted, there are no second chances. Young people with AIDS spend much of their time trying to fight the disease while coming to terms with dying.

This is a book about young people with AIDS—people who perhaps are very much like you or remind you of someone you know or have met. Many appear as unlikely targets of the disease, but it happened to them nevertheless. While other young people look forward to their future, these teenagers face an illness from which no one has ever recovered.

As their individual stories unravel within these pages, they've allowed us to see what their goals and dreams might have been before AIDS erased their plans. Also included is some important information about the disease—how it strikes and destroys bodies and lives, and what you can do to protect yourself.

Special thanks go to the wonderful people at Hope House and the Helping Hand Project, whose words and caring are shared throughout this text.

Karen S. was a fairly tall teenage girl with long auburn hair. Because she had large, sorrowful brown eyes, her parents and brother nicknamed her Bambi. They'd started calling her that when she was about six years old, but the name stuck.

Since her family had moved a number of times during the academic year, Karen had continually been forced to adjust to new schools and new people. She described this aspect of her life as being more work than school. Karen confided that by the time she was twelve, she'd decided that when she had a family of her own, they'd never move from their home for any reason.

KAREN

"My father has the kind of job where he's frequently transferred to new work sites. We'd lived in eight states by the time I'd turned twelve. I always envied the kids who grew up in one house. I thought it would be wonderful to have memories of spending Christmases with old friends or even graduating with the same group of kids you went through school with. As it is, my scrapbook looks something like the bulletin board of a travel agency.

"Our last move was the hardest for me. My father was transferred from Colorado to Connecticut after having been at the same place for nearly two years. For our family, that's practically a record for staying in one place. What made it worse was that we were leaving the best place we'd ever lived.

"My last school was really good. I liked my teachers and, although I'd never been the world's greatest student, my grades had begun to improve. Things were good socially too. I'd never been without a steady boyfriend for almost the whole time we lived there.

"The new school in Connecticut was different. The kids all had their little groups and they weren't too open to a newcomer. It was hard starting all over again, but I knew I didn't really have any other choice. Fortunately, my two best friends from Colorado liked to write. Finding their letters when I got home from school were the high points of my week.

"I'd been trying to keep my spirits up. But everything changed when I received a disturbing letter from my friend Gabriel. She wrote that there had been a big scandal at my old school. Ken, one of the popular guys at school, had been sick for a long while. When his condition worsened, the truth had come out. Ken had AIDS.

"My eyes followed the flow of Gabriel's writing easily. But even as I stood clutching her lavender stationery in my hand, I could feel my knees start to go weak. It was incredible to even think that Ken could have AIDS. He had been on the football team and was quite a macho man at school.

"A while ago there had been rumors that he and some of his friends had been into drugs. But I didn't believe it. Ken never looked like he'd been on anything. And who'd think a school star like that would be stupid enough to get involved with needles. Still, if he had AIDS, he probably did. That had to be the only way.

"I had dated Ken for about five months. He was in with the real popular kids, and I was thrilled when he showed an interest in me. He was the only guy I ever went out with who was on the football team.

"I hadn't planned to sleep with him, but I did. Ken was very persuasive, and I think I wanted to believe that he liked me much more than he did. About two months after we started having sex, Ken broke off with me.

"At the time, it hurt because I'd needed to believe that I had really been someone special to him. Ken started dating another girl right away. I didn't think that I'd ever go out with anyone again. But within a few weeks, Chris, the school newspaper's editor, asked me out. Chris wasn't on the football team, but he was really cute. We found that we had a lot to talk about too. We started going steady, and I was still seeing Chris when my dad announced the big move to Connecticut.

"I tried to tell myself that what happened to Ken wouldn't affect me. I had heard somewhere that not everyone who has sex with someone who has AIDS catches it. Still, I knew the odds were stacked against me.

"I kept hoping that I'd slip through the cracks. I hadn't been a bad person. I didn't deserve to die. And even though Ken had dropped me, I didn't want him to have AIDS either. Yet Gabriel had written that he didn't have long to live.

"I tried not to think about Gabriel's letter. But a few months later, I caught a cold that just wouldn't go away. I began to lose weight and I always had a bad sore throat. There were many nights when I'd wake up in a sweat.

"My parents were concerned. They wanted me to see a doctor. But I was too scared. I was afraid to tell my parents what I thought might be happening to me.

They didn't know that I had ever had sex with anyone. If they found out that I had done it with a boy who had AIDS, they'd be mortified. I didn't want to go for the test. I didn't think I could stand to hear the doctor's diagnosis.

"I tried to go on with my life. That wasn't simple, considering how bad I felt. I had to pretend to be better for my parents. But sometimes I was too sick to get out of bed in the morning.

"Yet during those first few months, I always pushed myself. I made my life a masquerade of smiles for my family. Whenever they said that I was getting too thin, I'd tell them I was dieting to look more fashionable.

"In the meantime, my stabs at making new friends at school came to a grinding halt. Most of the time I felt too lousy to put much effort into trying to be sociable. Often just being able to get through class was an accomplishment. I didn't tell my parents that I was too sick to go to school, because then they'd make me go to the doctor, and there was no knowing what that could lead to.

"I guess I wasn't a very good actress because a day didn't go by when either my mother or my father didn't ask me how I felt. I had the usual excuses ready for them, '. . . I'd really been busy at school, and I was just tired' or 'I was planning to stop dieting.'

"However, it wasn't long before my mother began to piece things together. She had also been corresponding with her old friends from Colorado. One of the women had written to her about the scandal at the high school involving the handsome football player with AIDS. The woman writing to my mother hadn't known that I'd gone out with Ken, but my mother recognized his name immediately.

"On the day this letter arrived, my mother confronted me as soon as I got home from school. Standing in the doorway of my room, she thrust the paper in my face and said, 'Well, Karen, I just hope this isn't why you look so terrible.' There were tears running down her cheeks as she spoke.

"My parents were not about to stand for any more nonsense. They wouldn't listen to excuses at this point. The next day I was taken to a doctor. By the end of the week, the test results confirmed that I had AIDS.

"My parents had always prided themselves on being practical people. Right off, certain steps were taken in our home to protect the other family members. I could only use the bathroom in the basement. I wasn't permitted to eat using the family dishes. Paper plates and plastic utensils were bought for me instead.

"Our housekeeper had been with our family since before I was born. She had traveled with us through all those different states. I guess my parents thought that they could trust her. They hoped that she'd be there to help them care for me. But the day she learned that I had AIDS, she quit. I remember her telling my mother, 'You don't pay me enough to die.'

"That's how the people I had been close to reacted to my illness. This continued in spite of the fact that two doctors and a public health nurse told them that AIDS cannot be transmitted through casual contact. It didn't help. Nothing helped. They were too scared to be smart.

"Meanwhile, my health continued to worsen. I couldn't go to school anymore. My parents had heard about the outrage Ken's getting sick in Colorado had produced. They didn't want to become well known for the wrong reasons. My parents said that my having AIDS could hurt my father's position in his corporation. My mother and father arranged for me to learn privately at home with a tutor who worked out of a special unit with the school.

"The arrangement seemed to work well for most everyone involved. The school was spared a controversy and my parents were spared notoriety. Unfortunately, the setup also spared me any real contact with other kids. I knew that was secondary in most people's minds. But when you know that you're going to die, it's not secondary.

"Not being isolated or cut off from everybody else probably becomes the most important thing in the world to you. My parents didn't seem to want anything to do with me now. I knew that they were caring for me out of a sense of obligation. I felt that if they could, they would have thrown me out of their lives. It was like fifteen years of love, closeness, and common experiences had never existed between us. They couldn't acknowledge that I didn't have long to live because they were so angry at me for getting AIDS. They might not have wanted me to be their daughter just then, but there wasn't very much that any of us could do about it.

"It's hard enough being in a new town without many friends. I know that I am not going to live out my natural life span. And it hurts too much to lose everyone important ahead of time like this.

"My parents had wanted to keep my illness quiet. But the word got out soon enough. Not one person from my school besides the vice principal and my English teacher came to visit me. A few people sent get-well cards, being careful not to mention what was actually wrong. But that was it. By the time of my first hospitalization, even those few niceties were over.

"As the illness progressed, the pain increased. I

was in and out of hospitals. We had heard about some new drugs for people with AIDS, but I never got to try them. The doctors said that the drugs were still somewhat experimental and that the best one only worked for certain types of patients.

"We also heard about another drug that was legal in Mexico, but still not available here. Somehow people were getting it from across the border, but I never got a chance to try it.

"I hated being a hospitalized AIDS patient while I was still well enough to realize what was happening around me. I was put in an AIDS unit, where patients with AIDS were grouped together. On an AIDS unit you are surrounded by dying and very ill people. Everywhere you looked, you could see what you might be like in the months to come or what you were a few months ago.

"Being hospitalized this way made it harder to even momentarily escape from an inescapable disease. It was a matter of being isolated again. There was no reason why we had to be grouped together like that. Since AIDS can't be caught by casual contact, why couldn't we have been mixed in with the other patients? It might have made things a little easier to be in a room with a girl my age who had simply broken her leg on a ski slope. Staying in the AIDS unit never let you forget who you were or what was going to happen to you.

"The disease did its damage to my body. It attacked my central nervous system. I had trouble walking and my vision worsened. As you can hear, my speech is slurred. I never used to sound this way.

"I was too sick to continue with the tutor. The end result of AIDS was becoming more obvious. I couldn't concentrate on school work any longer. Besides, I saw that the tutor was uncomfortable watching me deteriorate.

"It was plain that he didn't want to be around me by then. He surely wouldn't be the one to teach me how to say good-bye, without already missing everybody and everything so much. I needed someone to help me with that. But my tutor avoided anything personal. He stuck strictly to math and science.

"Summer came. I spent my favorite season in a wheelchair wrapped in blankets. Even though I wore thermal underwear and several other layers of clothes, I was still always cold. There were days when I felt chilled to the bone. I just couldn't get warm. I'd sit there shaking in my chair or bed.

"My father's feelings toward me worsened. I could tell. First, he blamed me for having had sex with Ken. Then he blamed me for getting sick. And now he was blaming me for dying in front of the family and ruining their summer. He just can't see that I don't have any control over the situation. I didn't want this to happen any more than he did.

"My father wanted to take my mother and brother on an extended summer vacation. I overheard him and my mother fighting about it one night. My mother said that I was too weak to be left alone, and that it would be difficult to find someone to care for me. My father wanted me to go back into the hospital. But my mother reminded him how few beds were available for AIDS patients and how acutely ill you had to be to win one.

"It ended up with my father and brother leaving for a month. My family had rented a summer cabin in upstate New York and that's where they went. My mother had firmly refused to go. She remained behind with me. I remember that she told my father that too few months were left. Her meaning was clear.

"So I spent most of the summer alone with my mother. She had to work very hard during that period. My coordination had worsened—I was barely able to get out of bed by myself.

"That July I turned sixteen. My mother baked a cake and brought it up to my room. Her eyes were wet. I guess we were both thinking that this would be my last birthday. I didn't even have the strength to blow out the candles. She did it for me.

"This year my mother decorated my cake differently. Usually, it had the correct number of candles on it for my age and one extra for good luck. But instead, this cake was filled with different-colored candles. It looked beautiful and aglow. Maybe my mother was trying to celebrate a lifetime of birthdays with me."

Author's Note: Karen died about three months after her interview. Her father was out of the country on business at the time of her death and did not return for her funeral.

Facts about AIDS

What is AIDS?
AIDS (acquired immune deficiency syndrome) is a progressively severe weakening of the immune system. AIDS damages a person's ability to resist and fight disease. People with AIDS become highly susceptible to infections and certain types of cancer. At this time there is still no cure for AIDS.

How widespread is AIDS?
AIDS has reached epidemic proportions. In addition to those who have developed the disease, at least a million more people have been infected. Those involved in AIDS research now believe that up to 99 percent of these individuals will come down with the disease as well. Up to ten million people may already be infected worldwide.[1]

*Allen is an extremely creative
young person who has demonstrated
ability in both art and music.
He is an accomplished flutist,
and one of his watercolor paintings
won second prize in a county-wide
art competition for high school students.*

*Although Allen claims he was aware
of being different as a very young
child, he didn't come to terms with
being gay until he was a junior
in high school.*

ALLEN

"I've been hospitalized three times so far with AIDS. I'm certain that I'll have to be admitted again. Each time I dread it. It's not just the discomfort and the endless tests. It's the humiliation that so many AIDS patients have to endure when they walk through that hospital door.

"AIDS patients are treated as second-class citizens. And if you're a teenager with AIDS, you can forget it. Then nobody thinks you deserve respect. Doctors, nurses, and other hospital staff should understand about illnesses. But when it comes to AIDS, they can be as condescending and cruel as someone who is completely ignorant of the disease.

"Often they are unable to accept that people with AIDS are angry over what's happened to them. Sometimes their attitudes seem to say, 'You're responsible for getting yourself in this mess,' rather than 'What can I do for this patient?' or 'How can I help him through the pain?'

"To make matters worse, there are numerous small indignities to bear. Once a technician was called into my room to fix the heating unit. He didn't need to go near my bed, but that didn't matter to him. He came in carrying a tool box and dressed in a surgical gown, gloves, and protective headgear. There he stood. An electrician who looked more like a spaceman. On another occasion, a hospital orderly stood outside the door and said loud enough for me to hear, 'Is that the room where the gay guy is?'

"The hospital publishes pamphlets about how AIDS is transmitted. Yet from the way their staff acted, you'd think they hadn't read their own materials. My mother spent nearly all her waking hours in the hospital with me. She felt she had to. As I became incapacitated, she acted as my voice. She fought for my needs when those in charge ignored my requests.

"People with AIDS are routinely treated differently than other patients. The nurses tend to downplay their suffering. An AIDS patient may have to press the buzzer several times before a nurse will come to ask what is wrong.

"We saw this happening while other patients were responded to immediately. The hospital staff tried to enter our rooms as infrequently as possible. At times, if you didn't keep ringing for them, they'd just let you lie there alone. If you have AIDS you need medical attention as much or perhaps even more than the next patient. On top of everything else, you shouldn't have to worry that the nurse isn't going to show up with your pain medication.

"During my last hospital stay, my mother remained with me from the beginning to the end of visiting hours. It was important to both of us that she be there. She is a healthy, capable woman who knows how to make herself heard.

"It was tough to watch her leave in the evenings. I knew that after she'd gone, no one would want to help me, no matter how bad things became. There were even fewer people on the night shift than on the day staff, and helping the AIDS patients was not their top priority.

"At least I had my family while I was sick. I hated to think about the other AIDS patients. Many of them were young and had been abandoned by their parents. Whenever my mother or father was at the hospital, they did as much as they could for them. But my parents weren't there twenty-four hours a day, and they both wanted to spend as much time as possible with me. My doctor doesn't think that I'll live out next year.

"I've already watched Jon, my hospital roommate, die of AIDS. I think that being with an AIDS patient at the end is one of the most difficult tasks any family or friend may ever have to face. Jon never lost his mental faculties as many people with AIDS do. We were able to communicate with him nearly up until he died.

"But, unfortunately, at times his pain became almost unbearable. Jon was given morphine to help him stand it. The medication was administered every four hours. And during the last hour, Jon would lie flat on his back, gritting his teeth, and clutching the sides of the bed with his fists. He was trying not to break down. He didn't want to give in to the pain that attacked his body. But he was defenseless against what was happening to him. Jon went through some very rough times.

"Jon's sister brought him his old teddy bear, Jeremy. It was just a battered wear-worn bear that Jon hadn't seen since he was about five years old. Jon outgrew Jeremy, but the old stuffed toy was never thrown away. His mother told me that she hadn't been able to part with Jeremy. She'd kept the bear in a toy chest in their basement.

"Jon's sister thought her brother might enjoy Jeremy's company again. She was right. Even after Jon threw out all the magazines brought to him and didn't want to watch television or listen to music any longer, he clung to that old bear.

"But a week before he died, he handed the stuffed animal over to his mother and said, 'Mom, take Jeremy home for me, will you?' She told Jon to keep the bear with him, but he insisted. He just said, 'I know that you'll take care of him. He'll be all right with you.'

"Jon's mother began to cry. As I turned away in the next bed, my eyes were wet as well. That was the first time Jon had ever openly admitted that he wasn't always going to be around.

"Then about three days before his death, I think Jon tried to say good-bye to all of us. He began planning a trip that the whole family was to take together. He wanted me to come along too. We were to go to Australia. We'd fly there first class. For the first time in years, his father would be able to get time off from work to enjoy a vacation.

"We'd have a wonderful time. There'd be cookouts, swimming, and camping. Jon couldn't stop talking about all sorts of things. He described how we'd photograph koala bears, kangaroos, and crocodiles. That's all he talked about all day.

"It was a strain on everyone. Jon's family knew he was dying. There'd be no vacation. And I certainly

LIBRARY
BRYAN COLLEGE
DAYTON, TN 37321

wasn't in shape to go anywhere. But to please him, we tried not to contradict anything he said.

"Jon was persistent. During the afternoon, he insisted that his mother go home to bring his large gray suitcase back to the hospital. She was happy to do it. She knew that she wouldn't have many opportunities left to do something pleasurable for her son.

"She brought Jon the suitcase and told him it was packed with everything he'd need for the vacation. He asked her to put it under his bed. Then he spent the rest of the afternoon with me, mapping out the details of our stay.

"That night, after his mother returned home, Jon called her from the hospital. He said that he knew that the family wouldn't be taking a trip, but that soon he'd be leaving us. That was the closest Jon ever came to openly saying good-bye. That was also the last conversation Jon ever had with anyone. That night he slipped into a coma. He died three days later without ever regaining consciousness.

"Jon had become my friend. It hurt to lose him. His death makes me think about what's going to happen to me and what it must be like to die. Sometimes, I wonder if I'll see Jon in heaven. And if we'll travel together there."

Facts about AIDS

How is AIDS transmitted?

There are a number of ways in which AIDS may be transmitted. Among them are:

Sharing body fluids through sexual intimacy. Mucous membranes exposed to blood, semen, or saliva allow the AIDS virus to enter the bloodstream.

The AIDS virus can also be transmitted through blood or blood products. This poses a special danger for intravenous drug users who share contaminated needles. AIDS can be transmitted through small undetectable drops of blood left on the equipment. Sharing needles and other drug equipment has significantly contributed to the rising number of AIDS cases.[1]

It is also important not to share razors or toothbrushes. At this time, there have been no reported cases of transmission in this manner. However, blood left on a razor through nicks or cuts, or on a toothbrush from vigorous brushing or bleeding gums could still carry the virus.

Is AIDS very contagious?
Unlike such diseases as chicken pox, flu, measles, and the common cold, AIDS cannot be transmitted through casual contact. It cannot be transmitted through sneezing or coughing. There are also no reported cases of AIDS transmission through using the same kitchen utensils, dishes, silverware, or drinking glasses. This is probably because the AIDS virus does not survive well outside the body.

AIDS is not transmitted through air, food, or water. It cannot be caught from a public drinking fountain or toilet seat or by eating in a restaurant. A waiter or waitress with AIDS could not transmit the virus to you by touching the food or breathing on it.

AIDS cannot be caught at a public swimming pool, as the chlorine in the water would destroy the virus. Even living in the same house as a person with AIDS or being around someone with AIDS for an extended period of time does not pose risk of infection, as AIDS is not transmitted through casual contact.

While it is true that the AIDS virus has been isolated in the saliva of infected patients, the disease has not been transmitted by kissing. This is because saliva only carries a minute amount of the virus. Dental instruments have also not been directly tied to the transmission of AIDS. This is because the virus would be killed by the standard sterilization procedures employed by dentists. Nevertheless, dentists have been directed to take proper precautions involving cuts that could result in a direct exchange of blood.

§& §& §&

Jackie is a short, slimly built
young girl with a painful past.
Although she dropped out of school
when she ran away from home,
Jackie is street smart. She has
an uncanny ability to see through
complex situations that enables
her to immediately get to the
core of matters. When asked
what she'd like most for herself,
Jackie answered, "I wish that my
life could have been different,
completely different."

JACKIE

"When you're on the street, you hear all this stuff about AIDS prevention, but you don't listen to it. You can't. You don't think about the future. You don't want to, 'cause it might be as bad as the past. Or as awful as the day you're just trying to get through.

"Guarding against AIDS when you're out there all alone doesn't mean much. It's about as real as that 'Just Say No To Drugs' thing. I bet it's easy to say that from the White House, dressed in a beautiful gown and wearing all kinds of jewelry.

"How hard is it to say no to drugs when you're drinking champagne or eating caviar with important people from all over the place? Try saying no to drugs when you have to pose nude all afternoon in front of a bunch of stinking, raunchy old guys with cameras.

Most of those jerks don't even have film in their cameras. Who do they think they're kidding, anyway?

"If you have to sell your body half the time just to keep alive, AIDS prevention isn't foremost in your head. Getting through the day is. Or sometimes it comes down to getting through the hour. It's funny. Because there've been times when I didn't feel like going on any longer. But I always felt that the decision was mine to make. I never pictured what my life would be like if I ever got very sick. At least before, my life was still my own.

"But AIDS changes all that. You lose control. The disease takes over your body. You face a death that's even more horrible than your life was at its worst. And there's nothing you can do about it. There's no getting better now.

"I felt rotten for a long time before I finally went to the clinic. Nobody on the street really takes good care of themselves. Usually, you just wait for whatever's wrong with you to go away. There's a lot of pain in living that kind of life, so you try to forget what's bothering you and just look forward to those good moments when all the pain and unhappiness seems to lift. Of course, that was before AIDS. Before the real pain began.

"I was sick for months before I took the test for AIDS. Something had to be wrong with me. My legs ached badly even when I wasn't walking or climbing up stairs. There were days when I thought that they'd give out on me. I was nauseous a lot and I had these horrible headaches. Sometimes it hurt real bad. I felt as if my head was going to explode like a Fourth of July firecracker.

"It's scary to be sick when you're alone and don't have money. And that's where it was at for me. I thought that my boyfriend wouldn't want any part of me if I couldn't work the streets and bring him money. And I was right about him. Whenever I said I was sick and couldn't work, he'd say that I was lazy or stupid and good for nothing. Then he'd throw me out of the apartment. I don't know for sure if he thought I faked being sick or if he just wanted to get rid of me if I couldn't work.

"Once you're diagnosed as having AIDS, nothing's the same. All the bad feelings you had before seem worse. It's not just that you're going to die. It's more that you're going to die slowly and painfully. You have to face the fact that people are going to stay as far away from you as they can.

"Like when I told my boyfriend that I had AIDS, he said to keep away. He asked me if I were trying to kill him or something. Next I called my mother. That was even worse. I don't know why I did it. I shouldn't have expected anything. I left home when I was fifteen. My mother's new husband never wanted any of her kids around. To him, we were just excess baggage. The quicker we faded away, the better he liked it.

"It was a mistake to call her. I felt bad about it for weeks afterwards. My mother said that Pete, her husband, didn't want me to come to the house. And he didn't want her to see me either. He was afraid that somehow he'd get AIDS.

"What could I do? AIDS doesn't go away. I can't call back when I'm better. With AIDS, there is no getting better.

"Since I've learned more about AIDS, I think it's a miracle that I didn't get sick sooner. I did all the wrong things. I had unprotected sex. I took IV drugs. I slept with IV drug users. I know I shouldn't have lived my life so carelessly. But I can't go back and change things now. Besides, I used to think that only homosexuals got AIDS. I thought that if you weren't gay and especially if you were a girl, then you'd pretty much be safe.

"If you've got AIDS and you've lived on the streets, you're treated as a nonperson. While I was in the hospital, I met this lady who takes in babies and children with AIDS. She said that she knew what it must be like for me. She told me how somebody from her church had said that what she was doing for the little kids was wonderful, but that grown-ups with AIDS shouldn't be helped because they're getting what they deserve.

"Having AIDS can make you feel desperate. It's hard to accept that there's no cure for what you've got. When it comes right down to it, it's hard to accept that it's over for you.

"Believe me, I'm not dumb. I'm not waiting around for a cure or anything like that. If you've got AIDS, you know that there isn't any hope at this stage. The doctors and researchers spend their time looking for a vaccine to prevent AIDS. They're interested in saving those people who haven't been hit by the virus.

"I think that once you start to feel really sick all the time, you can probably count the months you have left. By then you're not much more than a living corpse. People with AIDS are just shocking reminders. You're there as living/dying proof. I think others are supposed to look at you and think that if something isn't done soon, what happened to you could happen to them.

"You hear about a lot of liberal big shots saying things like, 'What a shame nothing was done for those people.' But when you're one of 'those people,' the problem becomes very real. You can't escape it. You think about what's happening to you night and day.

"Having AIDS is like being inside a burning building. You're inside with a few others being burned alive. Your flesh is on fire. You hang out of the window and scream for help.

"Meanwhile, every now and then, you see an occasional fire engine and crew. But the truck speeds right past the burning building. Unbelievable as it may sound, the fire crews are heading elsewhere. They are checking the smoke detectors in the safe buildings. Making sure that the people who are still safe stay that way. And they're doing this while you and others are dying.

"If you even say the word AIDS today, people immediately think of the whole deathbed scene. They picture a weak and tired person who can barely lift his head. Somebody hooked up to wires and bottles and all kinds of machinery. That's probably how I'm going to die. But I can't face that just yet. I don't even want to think about it.

"There have been some people who tried to help me. A decent social worker at the hospital got me a place to stay in a special residence for people with AIDS. The people there are pretty nice and, at least with everything else that's happening to me, I don't have to worry about having a roof over my head. I'm grateful for that.

"But no matter where you are or who you're with, AIDS hurts. I get these terrible sores in my mouth and on my tongue. They blister, and sometimes my whole mouth feels like it's on fire. At times, I can't eat anything and it even hurts to swallow water.

"The other day I decided to call my mother again. Don't get me wrong. I didn't expect her to say, 'Darling, come right home. I love you more than anything in the world.' Like I told you, I'm not dumb. But AIDS changes the way you feel about your family or the important people around you. When you get this sick and you feel yourself starting to lose it, you know that you don't have a lifetime left to make up with them.

"I called my mother because I realized that pretty soon it'd be too late to ever change things between us. Like in six months, who knows if I'd even have the physical strength left to work it out with her. I guess I still love her. I'm not sure. But I know how great it would be to think that she really cared about me.

"As soon as she heard my voice, I could tell right off that nothing had changed. She didn't want to hear from me. So, at one point, I just came out with it. I said, 'Ma, don't you realize that I'm dying?' She said she knew that, but the truth was that everybody had to die sometime. She told me not to think negative thoughts. Then she said that she had to hang up because my stepfather had just come in and she didn't want him to know she was talking to me. As soon as she hung up, I remembered why I had left home in the first place.

"I spoke to my mother again a few months later. This time she called me. She said that she hated to bring up unpleasant things, but felt that she had to at this point. She was actually calling about my burial. She felt sure that since I was still a minor when I died, her and Pete would be responsible for my body.

"My stepfather had told her that they didn't have any extra money for funeral and burial expenses. My mother said that it wasn't right to expect them to foot the bill. She wanted me to call my boyfriend and have him send them some money for it. She said that it was only fair since she knew that I had made money for him in the past.

"I called my boyfriend to tell him what happened. A new voice answered the telephone. It was a girl's voice. After hearing what my mother said, my boyfriend reacted as I thought he might. He said that he didn't have any spare cash. Then he asked me if I thought he was my family or something.

"Sometimes, I think that nothing could be worse than what AIDS does to your body. Or the emotional hurt of knowing that you have a disease that's going to kill you. But thinking about how the people I loved really feel about me comes a close second."

Facts about AIDS

Are some people at high risk
of getting AIDS?
The groups listed below have been identified as being at high risk of getting AIDS:

Homosexual and bisexual men. AIDS has been especially prevalent among this group of individuals. They account for the majority of all adult AIDS cases reported in the United States.

Intravenous drug users. Female and heterosexual male intravenous drug users make up the second largest category of adult AIDS victims. This is an especially deadly area for women. The number of reported women drug users or women who have been infected by a male drug user has risen significantly in recent years.

Blood-transfusion recipients. Two percent of all adult AIDS cases are recipients of blood products contaminated with the AIDS virus. Recipients of AIDS-contaminated blood account for 15 percent of all AIDS cases among children.[1]

Heterosexual partners of high-risk individuals. Heterosexual partners of bisexual men or intravenous drug users are at serious risk of developing AIDS.

Hemophiliacs. Adult as well as young hemophiliac recipients of a clotting factor contaminated with the AIDS virus make up another high-risk group. However, according to the Food and Drug Administration (FDA), new techniques have now virtually eliminated the risk of getting AIDS from blood products needed by hemophiliacs.

Infants and children of high-risk parents. Most of the infants and children with AIDS have a parent who either has AIDS or carries antibodies for the virus.

&a &a &a

---

*Gary is a likable young man with
a spirit that won't be crushed.
As a skilled athlete, Gary had
excelled in swimming, baseball,
and track. Among Gary's goals
were plans to eventually become
a physical-education teacher and
to turn his younger sister into
an Olympic swimmer.*

GARY

"Three years ago I was in an automobile accident. My father was driving and I was alone in the car with him. We were riding along the highway when my dad dropped his cigarette. He only took his eyes off the road for a moment as he bent down to pick it up. But somehow he lost control of the car. We crashed into a steel lamppost on the side of the road. Somebody called an ambulance and we ended up in the hospital.

"My dad had a concussion. Otherwise, he was okay. But I had to be patched up. I needed a transfusion. Still, everything seemed to go along well enough then. The doctors and nurses repaired my body and I was out of the hospital in under three weeks.

"I recovered quickly. I was back in school in the fall, and by winter I was scoring points for my basketball team. I wasn't sick. I felt great. I had also met Tara.

She's probably the world's best-looking redhead. All in all, it had been a good year for me.

"Have you ever imagined what might be the worst thing that could ever possibly happen to you? What if somebody called you up and told you that you were going to die? And that if the people around you knew the reason why, they'd be afraid of you. Afraid of getting the terrible thing you've got. Sounds pretty awful, doesn't it? But that's just about what happened to me.

"The man whose blood was used in the transfusion after the accident had died of AIDS. The hospital then learned that prior to his death, he had been a blood donor. They also determined that I had been one of the recipients.

"The next step was an AIDS test. My parents kept denying that this could have happened to their son. They said over and over again that the test would prove that I didn't have AIDS. I don't know how many times they told me that I was going to be all right. My mother and father decided against telling my younger sister. 'Why worry her?' they said. Everything would be fine in the end.

"We felt pretty certain that my donor must have contracted the virus after he had given blood. It couldn't be otherwise. Medicine in America was too far advanced for that kind of tragic accident.

"Unfortunately, we soon learned differently. Things weren't going to go my way after all. And from what I've found out since, I'm not the only one. It happens much more often than it should. Blood screening is tricky. The system has not been perfected.

"I took the AIDS test at the hospital. It's a blood test. The test shows whether or not you have AIDS antibodies in your bloodstream. My test was positive. That means that the virus is in my system.

"Without knowing it, the summer of the accident I'd left the hospital with a death sentence hanging over me. The people whom I thought had saved me had accidentally killed me. I guess these slip-ups have to affect somebody. But you never think that somebody could be you.

"When I took the AIDS test, I looked and felt well. I had AIDS antibodies, which meant that I was carrying the virus, but it wasn't full-blown AIDS at this point. Although I knew it could happen. It could happen at any time. My immune system could start to fail. I could become especially susceptible to any terrible disease. And everyone knows that the life expectancy for people with AIDS is pretty short.

"In the meantime, there were more immediate difficulties to face. I had to keep my diagnosis a secret. Most people with AIDS do the same thing until they get so sick that they don't care anymore. If you had cancer or multiple sclerosis or something like that, your friends and neighbors might bring you food and flowers. They'd want to be there to comfort you. It's not like that with AIDS. You live your life surrounded by people who are afraid of people with AIDS. And you and your family learn to hide the truth.

"Every summer my friends and I swam at a local pool. There's some great-looking girls there. But last year some of my friends' parents decided that they didn't want their kids to go to the pool. They were afraid they would get AIDS. You can't get AIDS that way, but I guess that they didn't want to believe the facts.

"My parents tried to tell them it was okay, but that

didn't help. Eventually, my mom and dad were bullied into going along with the others. And my friends and I didn't go swimming in the community pool for fear of getting AIDS. It may sound funny, but when it was over, I felt ashamed of what I had done.

"At that point, I didn't know if I'd have a future. I'd been told that some people with AIDS antibodies never get full-blown AIDS. I might live a lot longer than someone who doesn't even have the virus. And I thought that a cure might be discovered before I showed any AIDS symptoms.

"Nevertheless, I had to put my life on hold. I couldn't get involved with Tara like I wanted to. I couldn't have the normal social life of a guy my age. All of a sudden, I wasn't supposed to love or want to be with a girl anymore.

"Tara didn't understand what happened. I've stayed far away from my dream girl. It hurt to even look at her at first. Everything we talked about or planned is finished. And I couldn't even tell her why.

"Tara was hurt. She couldn't possibly know what was wrong. And this was at a time when I needed her around me more than ever. But I couldn't say anything. And no matter how much I denied it, Tara thought that there was something else.

"No one knew for certain what would happen to me. At the time it was hard to think about what might be down the road. My grades dropped. My parents thought it was because I was worried. I can't say that I wasn't worried. I wondered if it were worth studying anymore. Would I still be well when it was time to go to college or get a job?

"Unfortunately, I didn't have to wait very long for the answer. A few months afterwards, I began to develop some of the early symptoms of AIDS. I started to lose weight. I had a bad cough that I couldn't shake, and sometimes I ran really high fevers.

"I've since been diagnosed as having ARC. That's the middle stage of the virus. You get some of the lesser symptoms of AIDS. We also learned that lots of people with ARC get worse. They develop full-blown AIDS.

"My family has refused to accept that things could get worse for me. They continually tell me to hope for the best. My father said that there are countless true stories of people who unexpectedly recovered. Patients, who to the amazement of the medical establishment, have overcome fatal diseases. People who managed to go on living even when they were supposed to have died.

"My parents hope that if they look for other types of cures, I'll be all right. I don't know if this is possible. But I hope so, and I'm certainly going to try.

"My father has talked to some doctors who have left traditional medical practices. These physicians believe more in natural cures. They told us that there is some evidence to suggest that massive doses of vitamin C may be effective in combating the AIDS virus. So I've been taking that.

"We also went to New York City, where we saw an acupuncturist. Acupuncture wasn't done on me, but he mixed a special compound for me instead. It's made from the ginseng root combined with other ingredients. It tastes worse than anything imaginable. But if it works, who cares?

"Some people with AIDS get a purplish rash on their bodies. It's supposed to be a symptom of one of the diseases which frequently strike AIDS victims. I haven't had the rash yet, but if I should get it, we're prepared. We found out about a solution that's supposed to help.

"It's a type of harsh car-cleaning solution which is to be applied to the skin. The solution acts as a skin irritant. It causes the skin to break out in a rash. But it supposedly also signals the body's immune system to go into action. The liquid serves as sort of an immune-system stimulant. The resulting body reaction is to make both the rashes caused by the fluid and by the disease disappear.

"My father is determined to fight this thing any way we can. In the spring my parents are taking me to a faith healer in Mexico who's supposed to have helped other AIDS victims.

"My regular doctor in the United States thinks that all this is a waste of money. He keeps telling us not to get our hopes up high. He said that any incurable disease is a field day for unscrupulous quacks who want to make a fast dollar off desperate people. He may be right, but I hope not.

"My parents say that they are willing to pay what-ever it costs to help me recover. They told the doctor that they don't want to be left with a dead child and money in the bank. Right now, trying everything to save my life is more important to them than assurances that they are spending their money wisely. We can't afford to be certain about everything we do. That's just the hand we've been dealt. When you have AIDS, you learn to take chances. There is no other choice.

"I want to beat this thing. I want to go on living. I'd give anything to have my old life back. Even if these alternatives help to keep me alive and feeling better for a little while longer, it will have been worth it. And if not, at least I'll know that I didn't give up without a fight."

Facts about AIDS

---

*Can you become infected
with the AIDS virus through
a blood transfusion?*
Presently, the risk of transmission through blood transfusion is extremely low. This is due to the fact that donated blood is now tested for the AIDS antibody. Donors are also screened for risk factors.

However, as much as six months to a year may pass before an infected individual develops detectable AIDS antibodies. Therefore, an infected person might unknowingly donate contaminated blood during this time that could pass into the general blood supply. For this reason, individuals in high-risk categories should not donate blood; they might unknowingly be in the incubation period.

Anyone who knows in advance that he or she will

need surgery requiring a blood transfusion may take a further precaution. Individuals may donate their own blood ahead of time to be used during their operation. This procedure is known as autologous transfusion.

*Does giving blood put you
at risk of getting AIDS?*
There is no danger of getting AIDS from giving blood at a blood bank. Each needle used for taking blood is new and has never been used before. As soon as the process is completed, the needle is destroyed, making it impossible for a blood donor to become infected with AIDS in this manner.

What is AIDS-related complex (ARC)?
ARC is an intermediate stage of the AIDS virus. The following are among the most common symptoms of ARC: Loss of appetite, weight loss, night sweats, fever, persistent dry coughing, white spots or unusual blemishes in the mouth area, weakness in the legs, swollen glands, diarrhea, and fatigue. Although ARC often develops into full-blown AIDS, this is not always the case. It has not been conclusively shown that a person with ARC will eventually develop AIDS. Usually the symptoms and ailments associated with ARC vary in frequency and severity among different individuals. However, generally, ARC is not life-threatening.

ə ə ə

Cheryl never wears makeup and her fresh-scrubbed face combined with her petite stature (she's just five feet tall) makes her appear younger than she actually is. However, there's nothing immature about Cheryl. She's learned to handle difficult situations well and has overcome some significant obstacles in her life. Although I met Cheryl while she was going through a serious crisis, she was wonderfully gracious. Cheryl radiates an unusual warmth that immediately puts people at ease.

CHERYL

"This time last year I thought I finally had my life pretty much in order. I can't say I had an easy childhood. My father walked out on us when I was six. That left me with a younger brother and an alcoholic mother. My father never sent us any money. My mother spent her days complaining about how horrible my father was. She'd hit my younger brother or me for no good reason or drink until she passed out.

"My Aunt Beck felt sorry for my little brother. He was her ideal child. She and my uncle already had two daughters, but they'd always wanted a little boy of their own. They live in this big, wonderful old house in North Carolina. They even have an orchard on their property. I've spent weekends there in the summer. It's a private paradise.

"When my older cousin went off to college, my aunt offered to have my little brother live with them. She told my mother that she understood how hard it must be to raise two children alone. Actually, I think my aunt had very little respect for my mother and the way Mom conducted her life. But my aunt acted sympathetically because she wanted my little brother, and she knew she'd need my mother's support to get him.

"As it turned out, getting my little brother wasn't difficult at all. My mother offered him up readily. She even suggested that they take me along with him.

"Unfortunately, my aunt declined the offer. She made some excuse about wanting to, but not having a big enough house. That's ridiculous. My mother and I were living in a one-bedroom apartment while my aunt and uncle had room to spare.

"But I had to face the truth. I was thirteen and my brother was six. I was skinny with stringy brown hair, while he had dimples and curly blond hair. He was young and sweet, while I looked gawky and awkward. Besides, my aunt and uncle had already had their fill of girls. My brother just had more kid appeal. So he left, and I stayed on.

"After a while, things turned uglier at home. My mom took up with a guy who, believe it or not, drank even more than she did. They were always angry and fighting with each other.

"I don't know why they stayed together. They weren't an ideal couple in any way. The only thing they had in common was blaming me for everything that went wrong. They were both unhappy people. Things always turned bad for them.

"After losing my brother, I hated living with my mother more than ever. At least before, we had each other. Now I felt alone. My mother or her boyfriend hit me nearly every day of the week. I wore scarves and hats to cover the bruises.

"I asked my aunt if I could stay with them for a while. But she said that it would be best if I tried to work out things with my mother.

"No one knew how to reach my father. It was strange—both my parents were alive, but I felt completely alone. I left home for good. I knew at that point that I really didn't have any family there.

"But being on your own at thirteen is no picnic either. I stayed with a whole string of guys who liked very young girls. It's hard to believe that there are men out there who are worse than my mother's boyfriend. But there are. And I kept finding them.

"I think that Larry was the most damaging one. He really messed up my head. Larry was a drug dealer. But he didn't tell me that until I was sold on him.

"At first he just said he was in sales. It didn't take long to find out the truth, though. There was always junk around the apartment. And all kinds of characters rang our doorbell at all hours of the night.

"Larry urged me to get high with him. The pressure and temptation were always there. I felt miserable, and soon I gave into it. He said that I wouldn't get hooked. But like just about everything else Larry told me, it was a lie. I was hooked. I wanted and needed Larry's drugs.

"I felt like a dog on a short leash. I couldn't leave Larry. Like a baby who needs a bottle, I needed the needle. I hated myself. I hated Larry. But most of all, I hated the drugs that I wanted so badly.

"I thought that it would never end. I thought I'd probably die a junkie. Hooked on trash and on Larry, who had kind of become my keeper. But it did end. The police busted Larry's operation. He was tried, found guilty, and I think he might still be doing time. I don't know for sure.

"Because of my age, I was turned over to the local social-service agency. The social worker there placed me in a residential drug-treatment center. Detoxing was awful, but I got through it. And I did well in the program.

"The counselors there were great. They seemed to really understand where you were coming from. I met Bill at the program. He was one of the counselors. Bill was wonderful. He was kind and sensitive and really cared about me. There was never anyone like him in my life before. We didn't actually become romantically involved until after I completed the program. He kept stressing that the most important thing for me was to get well and feel whole again.

"Things started to go better for me. Following the program, I moved into a halfway house. There was nowhere else for me to go. I got a job in a card store as a clerk. I went back to school at night. I wanted to get my high school diploma. Bill wanted that for me too. We had begun seeing each other and it was serious. Bill only wanted the best for me.

"I stayed at the halfway house for two years. I finally got my high school diploma. I worked with a counselor that was associated with the drug program. She helped me to work out some of the terrible feelings I'd carried around inside me for most of my life. I got in touch with my younger brother, who I hadn't seen in years. He was happy to hear from me and doing well. And incredible as it may sound, I forgave my mother.

"Eventually, Bill and I moved in together. Several months later, I became pregnant. The baby wasn't expected. But we loved one another and had planned to marry later on. Things just happened a little sooner.

"I could tell that Bill was going to be a wonderful father. He was great during my entire pregnancy. I worked in the card store until my eighth month, but Bill wouldn't let me do anything around the house. He made us terrific nutritious dinners because now he said he was actually cooking for three. Bill wanted a healthy beautiful baby.

"We moved to a larger apartment. It was a wonderful garden apartment. There was a small spare room for a nursery and a lovely garden out back. Bill and I found this adorable old-fashioned crib in a secondhand furniture store. We painted it white and tied rainbow-colored ribbons around the sides.

"We bought candy-striped wallpaper for the nursery. The paper had a teddy-bear border. When we finished, the room seemed marvelous. I think any child would have loved to grow up in that room. I know that I would have. And I was thrilled to have been able to have it for my own child.

"Bill and I took prepared childbirth classes together. I was careful not to take any medication. I ate mostly organically grown foods. I made sure that I watched my weight and got enough rest.

"We wanted to do everything right for this baby. I listened to classical music because I heard on a television talk show that babies are sensitive to sound before they are born. Bill and I got library cards, and we checked out stacks of baby books. We spent whole weekends discussing boys' names and girls' names. The baby wasn't even born yet, but Bill and I were already in love with the kid.

"Giving birth is not as much fun as buying baby clothes. I was in labor for nearly thirteen hours. But it was worth it. We had a beautiful girl. We named her Michelle. Everyone said that she looked just like her father. But I think she looked like me.

"I felt as though for the first time in my life, I had everything. A wonderful husband, a super baby, and a pretty apartment. Just everything. It was too good to last. And, unfortunately, it didn't last. When Michelle was just a few months old, we saw that she was becoming ill.

"The signs weren't good. The baby was too thin. She was losing instead of gaining muscle tone. Sometimes she'd run high fevers. Michelle always seemed exhausted. She didn't want to be played with like other babies. She hardly had the energy to stay awake.

"Michelle cried all the time. And the sound of her cries seemed to worsen daily. You could tell that she was a little girl in pain.

"Our pediatrician checked Michelle into the hospital. A number of tests were done on our daughter. I don't know how many times she was jabbed with hospital needles. Within a day, her little arms and legs were bruised from where they had drawn blood, given her medication, or put her on an IV. I remained with her whenever the doctors allowed it. But Michelle was still frightened, confused, and hurting.

"One of the blood tests done on Michelle was for AIDS. It showed that the baby was infected. My little girl hadn't cried for nothing. Michelle was dying. The doctors gave her less than two years to live.

"The medical staff took full case histories from Bill and myself. We were both also tested for AIDS. Bill was fine. But my test was positive. Even though I didn't actually have the symptoms of the disease, I was a carrier. I had unknowingly passed a deadly fate to my baby. I felt responsible for both beginning and ending my daughter's life.

"We traced it back to my days as an IV drug user. The most miserable time of my life had actually been worse than I knew. I feel like a walking time bomb. I can get sick at any time. My husband had escaped the virus so far. Yet if we continued as lovers, he could get AIDS as well. But the worst part was what had happened to Michelle. The most precious thing in Bill's and my life was being snatched away.

"We both felt shaken, but Bill took the news terribly. He blamed me. I don't see how he could, but he did. I hadn't touched drugs in nearly four years. Back then, AIDS was something new. Most people didn't know much about it.

"If I had had the slightest notion that I was a carrier of a fatal disease, I would have never had Michelle. I wouldn't have married Bill. I love them both too much to ever knowingly hurt them. I would have taken a test to find out if I were safe. But a few years ago, I don't even know if there was an accurate test for the disease.

"I went back to my former social worker for counseling. My whole world was coming apart. The social worker explained that Bill's cruel outbursts and his coldness were just his expression of rage over the situation. She promised that he'd work through it all. She thought Bill and I would be able to face this together as a couple.

"But Bill didn't change. Even though he knew that I never meant to hurt the baby, he blamed me for what happened to Michelle. My husband accused me of having been self-centered. Bill said that most people are able to cope without drugs. He added that my crutch had cost our daughter her life and put him at risk as well.

"Some days I couldn't believe what I was hearing. After all, wasn't Bill a counselor in a drug-rehab program? But I guess this time the situation was just too close to home. What Bill always seemed to forget was that I was carrying the virus too. The disease could strike my body at any time. And that was a separate terror I hadn't even begun to face.

"Bill couldn't forgive me. Instead of making up, he moved out. He continued to be Michelle's father, but he didn't want to be my husband now. Bill visited Michelle three nights a week. He took her to his apartment on weekends. And whenever she was admitted to the hospital for treatments, he was there too. But I could always see the disgust in his eyes whenever he looked at me.

"I lost my husband. I'm losing my child. And I may lose my own life too. Caring for a child who is dying of AIDS is especially hard. The nurses on the ward treat me like dirt. One even asked me if I were a prostitute.

"I'm home full time now with Michelle. The babysitter who used to watch her won't stay with an AIDS child. She's afraid of catching it. Some of our friends sent flowers and toys to Michelle, but none want to visit the apartment. I know they're afraid of being infected. But they don't admit it. They just say that they're busy.

"And, as if things aren't bad enough, the lease on our apartment is up in two months and the landlord has refused to renew it. He said he felt bad about asking us to leave. But he's afraid that he won't be able to rent the other units in the building once it gets around that 'AIDS people' live there. And the word on us is out. Our dry cleaner has refused to accept our clothes.

"I think what they're doing is illegal. But who has the strength or money to fight it? My landlord suggested that we move to another town. But Michelle's undergoing medical treatment here.

"Besides, how long would it be before we were found out wherever we went? When your kid has AIDS, people don't treat you like the mother of a dying child. Instead, you're viewed more like an escaped convict. Someone who should be locked away from other people.

"The problem is that your only crime was getting sick. And that could happen to anyone. If you have AIDS, you don't get a trial. No one is interested in hearing your side of the story. It's just easier to label you as garbage to be disposed of.

"You may have been a human being the day before your diagnosis. But once you have AIDS, you turn into a toxic waste problem."

Facts About AIDS

What is a silent carrier?

A silent carrier is someone who has been infected with the AIDS virus, but does not show any symptoms. It's been estimated that there are between one and two million silent carriers in the United States alone. These individuals test positively for AIDS. This means that the antibodies for the virus are present in their bloodstream. Silent carriers look, feel, and act as though they are in excellent health. It is important to note that although a silent carrier shows no symptoms, that person is still capable of infecting others.

Silent carriers have no way of knowing they are infected unless they are tested for the AIDS virus. It's impossible to say how long an infected person may remain symptom-free. At any time, these individuals can come down with ARC or a full-blown case of AIDS.

əð əð əð

---

*By the time I met Jason, he'd grown
extremely thin and gaunt as a
consequence of his illness. His
mother showed me a photograph
of her son that revealed a young
man who had once appeared strong,
handsome, and filled with vitality.*

*Jason is of medium height with
light brown hair and hazel eyes.
His hobby is photography; he had
planned to become a photojournalist
after completing his education.*

JASON

"When you have AIDS, you never make long-term plans. It's a way of protecting yourself. This year we had the family's annual Fourth of July barbecue at my aunt's house. It was a great day. Beautiful weather, barbecued franks, corn on the cob, and beefsteak tomatoes. I watched my cousins play volleyball, while the younger kids held relay races.

"People were nice enough to me. Everybody stopped by to chat. They could see that I didn't have the strength to take part in the sports, and I think they didn't want me to feel left out. My relatives were trying to be kind, but I could tell that they were guarded around me.

"There was warmth and smiles, but no hugs or kisses. I followed their cue. I didn't try to kiss them or get really close. I didn't want to frighten them or make them feel uncomfortable. I can't even count how many people I've sent flying off to rest rooms in the past to antiseptically scrub the spot where my lips had touched their skin.

"I couldn't help but notice how our usual Independence Day celebration had been changed since I got sick. For years, the party had always been held at my parents' home. But not now. No one wanted to come over any longer if they could possibly help it. And certainly no one wanted to eat off our dishes or use our silverware.

"Having the party at my aunt's house allowed her to control the situation. This year the get-together was held entirely outdoors. I didn't even have to enter their house. Only plastic utensils and paper plates and cups were used.

"When I finished eating, I was careful to place my own cardboard plate in the disposal can. At my cousin's birthday party, I had already caught my uncle scrubbing his hands with Ajax® at the kitchen sink until they were nearly raw because he had accidentally touched the side of my plate. It was just easier this way. I would spare him the fear, and us both the humiliation.

"As the party broke up, everybody said how great it would be when we were all together again for Thanksgiving. As might have been expected, that dinner wasn't going to be at my parents' home either. I tried to sound enthusiastic. But I couldn't help but wonder if I'd be in or out of the hospital at that point or if I'd even be alive. And I know that everyone else was thinking the same thing.

"But nothing was said. Nobody wanted to spoil the day. The hours with my family had slipped by quickly enough. I didn't want to think that my whole life was passing by at the same pace.

"I didn't know whether it was or not. With AIDS, it's hard to say how long you'll be okay between bouts. Or even if your life may be prolonged by whatever treatments are tried on you.

"When you feel better between infections, you try to rebuild yourself. You take whatever drugs the doctors order. You try to regain the lost pounds. People with AIDS become very thin. My family said I'd become all skin and bones. In fact, in Africa, they call AIDS the slim disease. Putting on weight when you have AIDS means eating even when you're nauseous, and then fighting to keep it down.

"My mother and father didn't want to talk about my having AIDS. It meant that they'd have to acknowledge that I was gay and that I was dying. And they couldn't easily do either.

"So as my immune system failed, it wasn't because I had AIDS. Instead, every time I became ill, the illness was seen as a separate sickness. I'd either get well or it would kill me. But AIDS wasn't the underlying cause. Not to them.

"When you have AIDS, you can't help but think about dying. There isn't a terminally ill person anywhere who hasn't thought about suicide at least once. Anyone who tells you otherwise is lying. Sometimes when the pain gets really bad, you just want it to end. It's then that you think you'd do just about anything to escape from the misery.

"I'd wonder about how to do it too. Would I be able to somehow get a hold of enough pills to go quietly in my sleep? Who'd help me? I can't picture anybody among my friends or family who could handle the responsibility or the guilt.

"I remember reading about a doctor who once helped a terminally ill woman to die. She would have died on her own within several hours anyway. Her physician just tried to save her from an excruciatingly painful last afternoon. She begged him to help her pass on. He gave her an injection and she died moments later.

"With that action, the woman's pain might have been over, but the doctor's problems had just started. He was reported to the hospital board by a nurse. He lost his license to practice medicine in addition to being tried and sentenced to a jail term. It must have been terrible for him. I don't think I'd ever want help badly enough to wreck someone's life and future that way.

"I heard about a man with AIDS who shot himself in the head. He was supposedly an older man whose family and friends abandoned him when they learned about his illness. That had to have been horrible. He must have been in a great deal of pain—both mentally and physically—to have gone through with it.

"I haven't actually thought about suicide in a long time. That's the strange thing about having an illness that's incurable. When you know that you're probably not going to live out your expected life span, every pain-free day seems so special. And when you're able to spend that time with the people you really care about, you feel as if you've put one over on the virus.

"Once you've been in extreme discomfort, you're grateful for the little things that most people take for granted. A day in which you can stop coughing for fifteen minutes at a time is like a trip to Disney World. And if you don't feel terribly nauseous or have chills, you begin to remember what it was like to be well.

"When you know you're heading downward, you

want to stop time. You see yourself wasting away, but there really isn't very much that can be done about it. You save whatever strength you have left to gear up for the medication and treatments you'll need to fight off each new infection.

"Any serious disease is awful. But if you happen to have AIDS, you lose everything at once. It's a double whammy. Sickness and stigma combined. The kids at my high school didn't know that I was gay. It wouldn't have been accepted there. I would have been treated as though I had AIDS before I ever became ill. I kept a low profile at school. The guys I went with were older.

"Officially, as of yet, we haven't revealed my true diagnosis to the people at school. As far as they know, I have cancer. That's at least partially true. I have Kaposi scarcoma, a form of cancer that most often strikes AIDS victims.

"I didn't have a lot of friends at school anyway. There were some kids who came to visit when I was first out of school. They were nice. We were all in the band together. But after a while, they stopped coming. I think it made them uncomfortable to be around a sick person.

"We had never been that close anyway. They may have put two and two together and guessed that I had AIDS. I know that there were rumors going around. But my family firmly denied them.

"My parents and I agreed that after it was all over, they would reveal the actual cause of my death. I thought it would probably make things easier for others who become ill as I did. But right now, my family could not take on both a cause and a dying son. It was just too much for them. Especially since they hadn't been able to accept who I was and the only life style that had been right for me.

"Although they had been shaken by everything that happened, my parents stood by me. The important thing to all of us now is my getting the best care, and keeping as many options open as possible. AIDS forces you to live in the present. You don't spend time anymore thinking about the future or a career. Your major daily challenge becomes trying to keep from throwing up your lunch.

"The wasting-away process that's part of AIDS is awful. Watching me lose so much weight was also really hard on my parents. Once my mother insisted that we go out to a very good Italian restaurant about twenty miles from home. She knew that I liked pasta dishes, and I think she was trying to fatten me up. When the waiter brought over my plate, the fettucini smelled delicious.

"But the good feeling didn't last. As I began to chew my food, the familiar wave of nausea swept over my body. I only hoped that I wouldn't puke right there at the table. I excused myself quickly to rest in the car while my parents finished their meal. I still remember the look on my mother's face as I raced from the restaurant.

"Bit by bit, I'm losing the battle to remain a complete person. I hated the idea of becoming an invalid. I didn't want anyone to have to take care of me.

"But as you become weaker, I know it can't be helped. Sometimes things get pretty bad. I ran high fevers, and nothing helped to bring them down. The fatigue was terrible. It seemed to creep all through me. Many days I just didn't have the strength to get out of bed. Sometimes, it took all my energy to turn over on my side.

"There were days in the hospital when I really had to fight going under. I had a lot of trouble breathing then. I remember how both my father and my mother stayed at my bedside trying to cheer me up with small talk. They remained with me all through visiting hours. One or the other never let go of my hand.

"Now I can't remember what they said. I only know that the sound of their voices made me want to go on. Without actually saying it, I think that we were all trying to keep away death. I really wasn't part of the conversation. At best, I could mutter a weak yes or no. Sometimes I'd just nod my head. I think that I must have kept fading in and out. But it didn't matter. I wanted to be there, and having my parents with me helped.

"So far I've lost nearly thirty pounds, and I wasn't overweight to begin with. I hate looking in the mirror anymore. I know my face looks like a skin-covered skull. Even with love and good medical care, the disease is punishing. You're left exhausted.

"When you're in the hospital for extended periods of time, you see people die. I shuddered the first time I saw a body rolled out on a cot with a sheet over its head. It's a frightening feeling. You try to stay away from the dead person's room. Or you find yourself avoiding the glances of the dead person's relatives when you pass them in the hall. I think in a way that you're trying to hide from death. You don't want to get too close to it. You want to try to stop it from reaching out for you too.

"There was one very sick person that I had sort of made friends with at the hospital. But one morning when I went to see him, I noticed that his bed had been stripped down to the mattress and that all his things were gone. I asked another patient I knew from the patients' lounge if my friend had gone home. He answered, 'No, he never made it home. He died last night. I'm right next door, so I know. I heard his sister wailing for him too.'

"When you have AIDS, you get used to hearing things like that. Your life becomes a series of highs and lows. People with AIDS sometimes have as many as two or three diseases at once. A lot of the time, you feel drained and shaken.

"Whenever you recover from an infection, you feel like you've won a war. Now you're able to look forward to people, music, and videos again. It's great.

"For a little while, you've been granted a pardon. You're on furlough from the disease. But feeling well doesn't last for long. You can't change the fact that your immune system is finished. You're just a sitting duck for the next germ. Before you know it, you'll be sick again. Then you'll push yourself to go on. But it makes it worse to know that one of these times, you're not going to recover."

Facts about AIDS

Isn't AIDS a homosexual disease?
Since, at the onset of the epidemic, the virus hit the homosexual community most heavily, many people thought of AIDS as a gay disease. However, this is incorrect. Both heterosexuals and homosexuals have contracted the disease.

Why are so many people
with AIDS homosexuals?
This may be partly due to the fact that the virus may be spread more easily through anal intercourse. Tender membranes surrounding the rectum are more prone to small cuts and tears through which the virus can pass. When this happens, the AIDS virus gains direct entry into the bloodstream.

Allison, who said that her middle name should have been "The Brain," had been an outstanding student ever since elementary school. In addition to retaining an exceedingly high grade-point average, Allison had won two school-achievement awards in foreign languages. Allison liked her French class best, while she tried to tolerate gym periods.

ALLISON

"It's still hard for me to believe I have AIDS. I'm not in a high-risk group. I've never done much of the stuff that gives you the disease. I don't do drugs and have never had a transfusion. So my doctors and counselor have narrowed down the cause of my illness to my sexual experiences.

"That's a cruel joke. Until last summer, I hadn't had any sexual experiences. I had never been overly popular with boys. The boys at school went ape over thin girls. The cute cheerleaders were the ones who always had the rides home after school.

"I, on the other hand, had been waging a lifelong battle with my weight. I'd lose the pounds, only to put them on again nearly as quickly. I never had a good figure. I'm just built very much like my father—short and stocky.

"I know I'm not a head-turner. I wasn't a hit with the boys at school. When everyone I'd asked found an excuse not to be my prom date, I had to pay my older cousin from out of town to escort me.

"Part of the bargain was that he had to lie about who he was. I made him tell everybody that he was my boyfriend who was attending college out of state. My cousin hadn't even been able to get into college.

"I never had sex with anyone until the following year. Because of my grades and involvement in extra-curricular activities, my application to become one of our school's foreign-exchange students was accepted. I'd be away from home for several months. During that time, I'd attend school in France as well as travel throughout Europe. I was great at languages and saw this as the chance of a lifetime.

"Things were very different for me in Europe. There I wasn't just an overweight brainy girl. I was seen as something special. I was someone exotic. And finally some older boys took an interest in me.

"I lost my virginity in Italy. When I did it, I thought I only risked becoming pregnant. And I had seen a doctor to get something to prevent that. I know now that birth control pills will not protect you from the AIDS virus.

"In Europe, I felt popular. I can't describe how wonderful it was to be desired and appreciated for the first time in my life. They didn't have this thing about being skinny. I was considered attractive. Now I didn't have to beg for a date—I was sought after.

"Maybe it all went to my head. Looking back now, I know I should have been more selective. But I never imagined that I was risking my life. I thought I was only dating. Besides, there are so many girls in the states who've had sex more often than me and are still in excellent health.

"My doctors have convinced me that one of the boys I was with had to be either an IV drug user or a bisexual. It's true that I didn't know any of them really well. There were also language barriers to deal with.

"In my mind, I've gone over all my dates with them a thousand times. I can't imagine any of them doing anything like that. But obviously, I'm wrong. Besides, I know that those are probably not the kinds of things a boy would tell a girl he'd just met and was trying to impress.

"So here I am. The girl who couldn't get a date got AIDS through sexual transmission. I know that the odds against my contracting AIDS were high. It's difficult to believe that I caught the virus from a European. AIDS is much more common in the United States than abroad.

"I've learned that no one is immune to this lousy, stinking disease. The AIDS epidemic has made easy sex prohibitive. Anytime a healthy girl gets an offer like that, she should stop and ask herself if it's worth the risk involved. The way the disease is spreading, I'd advise any girl to wait until she's married. Even then, she better have known the boy for at least ten years. In some cases, AIDS symptoms haven't appeared for seven years or longer.

"AIDS is a real dream smasher. I knew about AIDS before leaving for Europe. I'd even done a report on it. But I thought of the disease as being confined to high-risk groups. I was the girl who worried about getting a boyfriend. I never dreamed I'd be getting an incurable disease along with the loving.

"If I had syphilis or gonorrhea, I'd need a few

painful injections or perhaps a week's worth of pills and I'd be cured. I could start my life over again. If I drove too fast on a highway, I'd get a ticket. If I weren't involved in an accident, I'd have an opportunity to change my actions. At the very worst, my license would be suspended for a while. But AIDS denies its victims first-offender status.

"And that's why no matter how I try to look at things differently, I'm still angry at myself. How could I have felt so invincible when an epidemic is sweeping the nation? My counselor told me that unless a cure is found soon, there won't be enough hospital beds available in major cities for all the AIDS cases.

"Now there's no turning back. The disease never lets you forget it's there. It's a constant reminder that my future is over. It's not like being a pregnant teenager—a girl who made a sexual mistake. I can't have an abortion or give the baby up for adoption. My error in judgment isn't correctable. Am I a pioneer in a new category? A separate classification made up of a growing few? Teenagers who are dying because they had sex with the wrong person.

"My counselor says that there are no right or wrong people—only individuals with an incurable illness. I think it's easy for her to talk that way because she isn't dying. She has a lucrative future ahead of her counseling all of us who are. People with AIDS don't have very much to be excited about.

"One of the worst parts of the disease is the wall of secrecy that immediately goes up following the diagnosis. It's a necessary evil. In our society, having AIDS makes you an untouchable. It's bad enough that this virus wipes out the rest of your life. You can't let the stigma attached to it ruin whatever 'well time' you have left. Hiding the truth is almost instinctual. It's taking a measure of self-protection in a no-win situation. My older brother calls it survival camouflage.

"Once the news had settled, my family sat down together to decide how to handle things. We determined that no one outside our immediate group would know. We needed money now more than ever, with my diagnosis and my brother being away at college. My parents didn't want anything to threaten their jobs.

"Both my mom and dad are elementary school teachers. They don't have AIDS. But it wasn't hard to imagine a public outcry against their working with children. If you have AIDS, you learn soon enough that your family will often be treated as badly as you are.

"Having AIDS is hard. But having to pretend there's nothing wrong when you know you're going to die is probably the most difficult thing I've ever had to do. But I managed to stick to it. I was too aware of what would happen if I slipped up.

"I felt light-years apart from my two best friends. The three of us were like sisters. In fact, since none of us had a real sister, we used to pretend that we were related.

"We'd always told each other everything. Now, at the worst time of my life, I couldn't talk to them. I had to act as though I were still worried about getting an A in French and making it through the tryouts for the school play.

"When I had pneumonia, I pretended that it was just regular pneumonia. Nothing more. They had no way of knowing that the condition was an AIDS spin-off. I had to smile at my friends' assurances that in no time I'd be up and about.

"I began to avoid my friends. It was too hard to act optimistic around them when I was so scared of what might happen to me. The parents of one of my friends had been going through a divorce, and she had become the object of a bitter custody suit. In the past, I, along with my family, had been her support lifeline. But now I found that I didn't have much sympathy left to give.

"Maybe at the time I was mourning for myself. I'm not sure what was happening. I only know that I'm impatient. The things that were once important now seem annoying and trivial. I think I just hurt too much myself to show my friend the compassion she needs.

"The disease progressed. I became ill more often. I backed even further away from my friends. They couldn't understand why I felt so miserable most of the time. Some of the people at school suggested that I was taking myself too seriously. I had already missed too much school. Everybody was beginning to think I was a hypochondriac. It was hard to hear that and not respond—but what else could I do?

"It helped to have my brother around. He was kind and had managed to keep his sense of humor through all this. Having him close by was reassuring, but I didn't see him as much as I would have liked. My parents had always stressed the importance of education, but now they urged my brother to take a semester off from college to be with me. I think they sensed how much I needed him.

"But my brother decided to go back to school anyway. It was all right. I understood where he was coming from. When my brother was home, he had to lie to everyone around him, including me.

"How long can you ask someone you love to be 'on stage' like that? He was doing the best he could, but my brother needed a break from the pain. I think it was unfair to ask him to stay home to watch his kid sister die. So, as it turned out, it was largely left to my parents and me to keep up the charade.

"Of course, there was one place where we didn't put up a front. Everyone on the hospital staff seemed to know who the AIDS cases were. And as soon as you were labeled with AIDS, that's exactly what you became—a case—no longer a patient or a person in any sense of the word.

"In their eyes, you're automatically reduced to scum. They've already assumed that you're a drug addict. And when you're lying in a hospital bed with a tube stuck in your arm and another up your nose, you're hardly in a position to boast about your accomplishments.

"You don't have the strength or courage left to tell them that you'd been on the high school honor roll for two terms or that you play the violin beautifully. I don't think they'd be interested in hearing it anyway. It wouldn't fit their view of anyone with AIDS.

"I hardly knew those people, and I shouldn't have cared what they thought. But somehow it mattered to me. Stripped down to my hospital gown, I had nothing to show of my life but a medical chart that said I had AIDS. I felt naked without my report card or any of the achievements that had always given me a sense of pride.

"Before long, I was continually in and out of the hospital. I'd go there for medication, treatments, and all kinds of tests. Whenever possible, my parents tried to care for me at home. But sometimes I'd get very sick. Then I'd be admitted to the hospital again and they'd try to make me well. When I improved, I was sent home to try to resume what was supposed to have been a normal life.

"AIDS can disrupt any family. It makes everyone

feel guilty. I think the people around me feel both lucky to be healthy and heartsick because I'm dying. I remember that my father always said that the worst thing that can happen to a parent is to have his child die before him. Parents were not meant to survive their children. It was unnatural. My father said the grief that comes from the loss of a child is immeasurable.

"My father is trying to be brave on the outside, but I can't help but wonder how he really feels. Out of everyone in my family, my father is the strongest in his denial of what will eventually happen to me. If he thinks I'm going to die, he refuses to admit it.

"Dad always has a pep talk on the tip of his tongue. 'We're fighters, aren't we?' he'd say. 'We're going to beat the big A. It's our family against the odds.'

"I've never believed him for a moment. But I think he'd be shattered if he knew that. So I act like my dad's brave young soldier whenever he's around. It's a hard role, and very often I just want to stop acting.

"I'm tired of feeling so bad and still having to please everyone. Sometimes I wish I could cry in my father's arms. I want to feel sorry for myself. But most days, it looks as though my father is taking this worse than me, so I have to act like an encouraging parent myself—full of positive energy and good cheer.

"My mother handles my having AIDS differently. She became bent on protecting me from germs. She had always tried to protect and shield me. Even when I hadn't needed her, she still always wanted to be in the wings.

"When, at the age of nine, I had finally insisted on being allowed to walk with my friends to school alone, she reluctantly allowed it. I'll never forget how embarrassed I was when one of my friends spotted her following us behind the bushes. She called it 'mother love.' My brother jokingly referred to it as 'smother love.' And when I got sick, her feelings of protectiveness snowballed.

"I think my mother blames herself for my getting AIDS. She had wanted to accompany me to Europe when I was on the exchange program. But everyone said that was ridiculous. I had to grow up sometime, didn't I? There were a thousand other reasons for her not to go. She couldn't get off work, we couldn't afford it, none of the other parents were going, etc. But I think she feels that if she had been there, I wouldn't have been with those boys. That's probably true. But I certainly never blamed my mother for what happened.

"Because my immune system is messed up, my mother is determined to ward off any germs that might cross my path. It's an impossible task, but no one can talk her out of it. For example, no guests with colds are allowed in the house. I think she might have already offended a few people as she turned them away and insisted that they take a raincheck.

"They didn't know I had AIDS. I can just imagine what they thought. But nothing seems to faze my mother. I can't pick up the telephone receiver without her taking a cloth with ammonia to it first. She tries to disinfect everything that comes near me. As a result, my mother creates a lot of busy work for herself. But she needs to do it. It's her way of coping with the situation.

"Sometimes, I'll feel good for weeks at a time. My father attributes it to my positive attitude. My mother stuffs me with health food and handfuls of vitamins.

She makes sure I stay away from crowds and out of drafts. Those weeks are the best times for us. Then we'd feel closest as a family.

"But beneath all the warmth and denial, we still can't forget that I have AIDS—a disease that no one has ever recovered from. My parents do their best to continue with their lives, but they needed help with this thing as much as I did.

"Because we all live with this deep, terrible secret, my parents missed out on the support and assistance friends can provide at a time like this. My counselor hooked them up with a support group of parents of children with AIDS. People participate in the group anonymously. They only use first names. Being together showed these people that there are others out there like them. The support group helped my parents, but they were still concerned about me.

"When they asked if there was a similar local group for young people with AIDS, my counselor told them that there weren't any at this time. The last such group fell apart because the group members kept dying, and the loss had a devastating effect on those left.

"Even in the best environment, when you have AIDS, you can't escape the painful truth that you are alone. And when the time comes, you'll have to die alone."

Facts about AIDS

What behaviors especially
put you at risk?
• Sex without a condom if there's a possibility that your partner could be infected. • Anal intercourse—whether or not a condom is used. • Sex with someone who has multiple partners or engages in other high-risk behavior. • Sharing needles and/or other IV drug-related equipment.[1]

Can using condoms reduce
the risk of AIDS?
There is no guarantee that using a condom can provide complete protection against AIDS. However, the use of condoms by sexually active individuals has been shown to significantly reduce the transmission of AIDS as well as other sexually transmitted diseases.

Is there a connection between
AIDS and drugs or alcohol?
Engaging in safer sexual behavior means using good judgment and acting maturely when making decisions regarding intimacy. The use of drugs or alcohol can cloud an individual's judgment and affect his or her ability to make prudent choices in important matters. Although drugs and/or alcohol do not transmit the virus, these substances may prevent someone from taking the necessary precautions to safeguard his or her own good health. It is also important to note that some drugs (alcohol, marijuana, and amyl nitrate, among others) tend to weaken the immune system.

Can you get AIDS from
a mosquito bite?
It's impossible to get AIDS from a mosquito bite. Unlike such tropical diseases as yellow fever, malaria, and others, AIDS is not transmitted through the mosquito's salivary glands. The AIDS virus is also not carried by other insects.

*Maria is an attractive teenage girl
with long dark hair. Being somewhat
of a loner, Maria claims she never
had many girlfriends.*

*Although Maria has always lived in an
urban environment, her dream is to
raise a beautiful child and reside in
a lovely home high in the mountains.
Maria said that if she had a garden,
she'd fill it with roses and lilacs.*

MARIA

"I tested positively for AIDS. I haven't felt sick yet. But I'm sure the results have to be correct because I took the test twice.

"I went to one of those clinics where you're tested anonymously. All you have to give is a first name. Actually, you could use any first name. Each person is assigned a number. They give you a time to call back. When you call back, you tell them your number and the date you were tested.

"Next comes the hard part. You wait on the line while they look up the results. They return quickly, but it feels like forever when you're waiting to find out. Then, if the answer is something you didn't want to hear, you wish that they never came back to the phone.

"My news wasn't good. I didn't want to believe it. I thought there must be some mistake. It can happen, especially at a large place like that where nobody knows who you are. So I took the test for a second time. When the results were the same, I had to begin to face the truth.

"The virus is in my system, or it wouldn't have shown up twice on the tests. But at this time, the disease isn't affecting me. I walk a thin line between good health and an early death.

"At first I didn't want to be tested for AIDS. I think I was afraid of getting a bad verdict. I used to date a boy who was on IV drugs. We were together for a while, but it's hard to be with a person on drugs for long.

"Drug addicts are possessed. Their need to get high is bigger than anything they could ever feel for you. They don't take care of themselves. And they don't have very much to give to another person. They're only sweet in-between times, while they're trying to get your money for their stuff.

"That's how it was between me and my boyfriend. I had just quit school about three months before and was working in a fast-food place when I met him. I still lived at home with my mother. I was never a good student and I'd hated school for years. I wanted to make some money.

"At sixteen, I told my mother that if she didn't let me quit, I'd run away or something. She didn't stand in my way. I think she knew how I felt.

"I went to work full time. A lot of good it did me. I fell for a good-looking guy who talked me out of nearly everything I made. I thought I could help him quit using drugs, but I ended up helping to support his habit. I couldn't stand to see him in pain. I know I was a pushover. But he had needle marks all over both his arms and legs. I didn't know what to do.

"Anyway, I guess he thought I wasn't doing enough. He left me to live in Chicago with an older girl. I think she probably had more money. It's hard to know. It hurt. My mother and the people at work kept telling me that it was for the best. He was always in trouble with the law.

"That was over a year ago. Since that time, I started seeing Tom. He's about two years younger than me and is still in school. He got me thinking about night school for myself. But a couple of months ago, I put all my future plans on hold. I found out I was pregnant.

"Tom's the father. But at fifteen, he's not ready for the responsibility. My mother wasn't too bad about it, though. She said that it was my choice whether or not to keep the baby. If I wanted to have it, I could stay home. She'd help me to care for her grandchild. And she said she'd make sure that I still had a chance to go to night school.

"So I decided to have the child. When you find out you're pregnant, you start to love the baby right off. It's just a feeling you don't have control over. Abortion may be right for some women, but not for me. Not now anyway. I wouldn't feel right about it.

"I was all set to go through with the pregnancy, but this AIDS thing kept gnawing at me. I couldn't change the fact that I'd been with a drug user for several months. My mother gave me a pamphlet that showed how you could catch AIDS from sleeping with someone like my old boyfriend. It didn't matter whether or not you ever used drugs yourself. The fact that I hadn't stuck a needle into my arm wouldn't protect me if my old boyfriend had the virus.

"I also knew that even if I carried the virus and showed no symptoms, my kid wouldn't be safe. I could still pass it on to my unborn baby and give birth to a very sick infant.

"Before I got pregnant, I didn't want anything to

do with AIDS testing. I think I was too afraid of what I might find out. Besides, I felt fine. My new boyfriend, Tommy, had been tested after he learned about my past. The test showed that he was all right. So, naturally, I thought that I was all right too. I knew it was still possible for me to have AIDS, but I didn't want to think about it.

"It was my mother who insisted. She said that I had to act right and start taking charge of my life. She was willing to help me care for a healthy grandchild, but she said she couldn't stand by quietly while I knowingly brought a child with AIDS into our home. My mother claimed that she didn't have the money or the emotional strength to handle it.

"At first I didn't know how to deal with what she said. I felt hurt and angry. We both cried and said some terrible things to each other. I asked her if it was fair to determine if you loved somebody by whether or not that person was sick. I guess I thought that maybe she wouldn't want me if I came down with the disease as well.

"I felt scared. My mother hadn't been married when I was born, so I never really had a regular family. But she had always loved me. She'd made a nice home for us. I'd been sure that my baby would do just fine with her and me. But now I didn't know if I could still count on her.

"After a while, things calmed down. And my mother explained how she felt. She told me that she'd never throw me out if I were sick. She realized that I had just made a terrible mistake in staying with my old boyfriend to begin with.

"But she said that the baby was another story. My mother believed that no one had the right to knowingly give birth to a baby whose only future was a short, pain-filled life. To her, it was unfair to have a child who'd only know suffering and death. Not if something could be done to prevent it.

"I respect her feelings, but I saw things differently. Even if I tested positively for the AIDS virus, there wasn't a guarantee that my child would be born with the disease. If the baby simply carried the virus, but showed no symptoms as I did, there wouldn't be any suffering involved. And maybe there'd be a cure before the kid ever got sick.

"If I had an abortion, I'd eliminate the possibility of my baby dying an early death. But then my baby would never be born at all. The child would never know any of the wonderful things about life. The kid would never hear music, or go to the beach, or build a snowman. He'd never taste ice cream, or pizza, or Chinese food.

"I want to have this baby. If the very worst happened and the child became ill, maybe by then better drugs would be available to help him. I tried to explain all of this to my mother. I reminded her that she hadn't aborted me, when someone else in her circumstances might have. I'm glad to be alive even with this AIDS thing. I want my baby to live too.

"But no matter what I said, my mother stood firm. She was still against my giving birth if I were carrying the AIDS virus. She said I had no idea of the responsibilities of motherhood. I had been a healthy baby, and our lives certainly hadn't been easy. A child with a terminal disease that would turn the whole neighborhood against us was just too much to take on. She urged me to take the test for AIDS. If I were clean, there was nothing to be concerned about.

"It was hard for me to schedule the test appointment. I thought the results might change my feelings about having the baby. It's one thing to imagine possibilities and another to face them.

"I had the test and you know what happened.

"I've tried to rethink the whole abortion thing. Maybe my child would be better off if he were never born. My mother's probably right. It's going to be hard for a kid to enjoy an ice cream cone if he's in horrendous pain.

"My mother has a friend who's a nurse. She told me that an infected mother has about a 50 percent chance of having a baby with AIDS. She took me on a tour of the hospital where she works and showed me all the infants with AIDS. Some of them had been abandoned by their mothers because they had the disease. They were alone in this world and very sick.

"I'm not against abortion. It's just that I always thought of it as being for people who didn't want their babies or couldn't take care of a child at the time of their pregnancy. But I want my baby more than anything. I'm willing to take care of the child, no matter how hard it becomes. I'm prepared to make whatever sacrifices are necessary. If that means putting off night school and taking a second job, I'll do it. I just want my child.

"My mother says that I don't know what I'm saying. She believes it's easy for me to talk big because I've always had her behind me. She's warned me that the wrong decision now could affect the rest of my life. She stressed that by the time I feel the misery of loving a dying child, it will be too late.

"I've thought long and hard about everything my mother and everyone else has said. But I'm still going to have this baby. I just hope my courage and health hold up. As long as I remain well, at least my child will have me.

"I understand that if the baby is sick, I won't be able to stay with my mother. I respect her right to protect herself emotionally. It's a little scary to think about being on my own. I've never lived by myself, and it's hard to imagine doing it with a sick kid.

"I know that there are homes for unwed mothers. You can go there to have your baby. Yet I don't think there are places you can live with a kid afterwards. Especially if the baby has AIDS. I don't know if anything is available. But I'm hoping that I'll never need to find out.

"So far, I've had a very easy pregnancy. I'm continuing to work at the fast-food place. I try to look forward to the future. It's hard, because sometimes my mother will look at me and cry. I don't want to know what she's thinking. I try to put those things out of my mind.

"I'm not sure of my future or what my child's life will be like. People with AIDS sit balanced at the edge of a cliff. Either we fall off or something more is done to help us. I'm hoping that we get the help."

Facts about AIDS

Can a pregnant woman with AIDS
pass the virus on to her unborn baby?
There is at least a 50 percent chance that a pregnant woman with the AIDS virus will infect her unborn baby.[1] The AIDS virus may be transmitted to the baby either before it is born or during birth. New mothers with AIDS can also infect their infants if they breast-feed the child.

Infants born with AIDS face an early death sentence. Unfortunately, in the United States, the number of cases involving infants and children with AIDS has dramatically increased. This is especially true in New York, New Jersey, and Florida. These three states account for the majority of AIDS cases among young people.[2]

*In Paul's hometown, his precision on
a skateboard had won him a reputation
as the neighborhood champion. Paul's
other passion is magic. As an amateur
magician, Paul put on shows for children
at the local hospital as well as at his
library. Paul's act was also featured
in his junior high school's variety show.*

*Paul has sandy blond hair and blue eyes,
and in the summer a blanket of freckles
covers his nose. Although Paul is very
fond of his family's two cats—Bread and
Butter—he wishes he could have a
dog like Spuds McKenzie.*

PAUL

"I'm a PWA—that's a person with AIDS. Most people say it's a crime that I have AIDS because I'm so young. But I think the real crime is that AIDS still exists as an incurable disease.

"My brother, Danny, was two years older than me. He died of the disease less than six months ago. He was a hemophiliac. So am I. Both of us had to have frequent transfusions. Our doctors think that we got AIDS through contaminated blood products.

"My brother became ill almost immediately. Our whole family moved shortly thereafter. My parents decided that we couldn't stay where we lived anymore. My brother and I grew up in a small town. Everybody knew everything about everyone else. That had never been a problem for us. We didn't have anything to hide. But AIDS changed all that. As soon as the diagnosis was known, it was time to get out.

"Our diagnosis was never supposed to have been public knowledge. Everything in our medical records should have remained private. We don't know for sure who started the rumors about what we had. My parents think it might have been someone who worked at the hospital or one of the receptionists in the doctor's office.

"Maybe whoever leaked it felt it was their duty to warn the town. Within weeks, my brother and I became the two most unwanted people in the neighborhood. We were suddenly a menace to the community. My father said that when his boys got sick, it was as if a natural disaster had struck town. I guess people didn't see that the real disaster was what they were doing to our family. In our neighbors' minds, having someone with AIDS next door was the equivalent of a tornado, a cyclone, or an earthquake.

"Even before we were diagnosed, it was obvious that most people in our town were afraid of getting AIDS. Our minister had described it as God's way of punishing the homosexuals for defying the divine word. He said we should still love and forgive these people, but that homosexuals were to blame for what happened to them. He had me convinced until Danny and I got sick.

"If we had AIDS, we knew for sure that what our minister said couldn't be true. My brother and I weren't homosexuals. We were both too young to have had sex with anybody. Now I think it's silly to believe that God would punish any one group of people by making them get sick and die.

"Where we used to live, the AIDS epidemic made it hard for anyone who might have been a homosexual.

I remember a man named Jake Barnes who worked as a short-order cook at the diner. He and his wife had split about a year ago. Although several of the women in town had wanted to go out with him, Mr. Barnes hadn't shown any interest in them.

"Maybe he was too hurt over what had happened with his wife. Anyway, at first he lived by himself in the big house he and his wife shared. Then about six months after she left, he took in a roommate. My parents thought that he probably needed help with the mortgage.

"But it wasn't very long before people began to whisper about him. They said that he was gay because he had a male roommate and didn't have a girlfriend. Everybody said that was probably why his wife had left him to begin with. To prove their point, they'd remark how he and his wife never had children, even though they'd been married for nearly three years.

"It was so unfair. People talked about Jake Barnes behind his back. They made jokes about him and called him a queer and a homo.

"But, once the AIDS scare began to spread, things really got bad for him. All of a sudden, people started to think of Jake Barnes more as a threat than just someone to ridicule. Because they thought he was a homosexual, they were equally sure that he had AIDS. Everybody said it was unthinkable for him to be employed as a cook in a local eating place.

"People pressured the diner owner to hire someone else. When he didn't act immediately, they stopped going to the diner. And Mr. Barnes was fired within a week. We heard that no one else in town would give him a job either. It was probably an unspoken agreement among the merchants. If the townspeople had planned to drive Jake Barnes out, they were successful.

Unable to find work anywhere, he left the county in under a month.

"My parents had seen what happened to Mr. Barnes, who probably wasn't even a homosexual and didn't have AIDS. They weren't willing to wait around to see how our neighbors would react to a family with two kids who really had AIDS. Even before everyone had heard the news, you could see that people were starting to act differently toward us.

"My brother and I were diagnosed at the start of summer. Danny and I were supposed to have gone camping with another family that had two boys about our ages. We had planned the trip three months ahead of time.

"But a few weeks before we were supposed to leave, our friends' parents decided that there wasn't enough room in the car for all of us, and that my brother and I wouldn't be able to come. It just didn't sound right. They hadn't bought a new car or anything. And their old car couldn't have shrunk.

"A whole string of similar incidents took place. Danny wasn't invited to his best friend's birthday party, even though every other boy in his class went. When my mother shopped at the fruit store, the manager rushed over to help her select what she needed. He had never done that before. I guess he didn't want her to handle the food.

"Nobody wanted to come over to our house anymore. All our friends were too busy doing other things to be with us. Yet we'd see them riding by on their bikes nearly every day.

"My parents played bridge with another couple on Thursdays. They had done so ever since I could remember. Now every week the couple found some excuse not to play. After a few weeks, my parents just accepted that the friendship was over.

"In some ways we were lucky. My father was a salesman with a good track record. He was able to get another job in a city up North. There were large hospitals there as well as other people with AIDS.

"It's hard for me to describe how Danny died, and what he went through before his last days with us. I get queasy just thinking about it, but I can't stop thinking about it. Danny was my brother. I loved him. Besides, I got the contaminated blood as well. What happened to Danny could possibly happen to me. I may die the same way he did.

"I've learned that AIDS affects people in different ways. Some people become very ill. Their immune systems seriously weaken. Then they usually catch one or more of what the doctors call opportunistic infections. Eventually, these illnesses kill them. The physical symptoms can be agonizing.

"But before the patient dies, AIDS can do something even worse to its victim. The AIDS virus can destroy a person's brain. This condition is called AIDS dementia.

"As of yet, doctors aren't sure exactly how it occurs. But they think that one of two things may be happening. The AIDS virus may directly infect the brain. Or the virus may disrupt the action of vital brain chemicals and the immune system. Our doctor told us that the brains of nearly 10,000 victims have been damaged either by the virus or by AIDS-related infections. Unfortunately, my brother Danny was among them.

"At first Danny just seemed confused. He'd get mixed up easily. He didn't know what day it was. Sometimes he wouldn't remember who his teachers were. We brought some of his favorite games to the hospital, but he couldn't concentrate long enough to play them.

"It wasn't long before Danny's balance seemed to go. He started bumping into everything. Sometimes when he walked, he'd have to hold on to something to keep from falling. Danny had been a great baseball player. It hurt to see him like that.

"As time passed, Danny grew increasingly forgetful. There were weeks when he didn't know where he was. Once, while lying in his own bed in our room, Danny cried for two hours and kept repeating that he wanted to go home.

"He had just been released from the hospital a week before, but obviously he didn't know where he was. Danny couldn't recognize the room we shared, even though it was filled with our stuff. My brother was either angry or sad much of the time. Nothing any of us said or did helped him to feel better. He was miserable. It was awful to watch.

"Toward the end, Danny went into his own world. We'd turn the television on to his favorite programs, but he didn't want to watch. He'd only stare at the ceiling and walls without saying a word. We all tried to talk to him, but he didn't seem to hear or understand us.

"You could see that Danny was in terrible pain right before he died. We stroked his shoulders and arms. Everyone tried to comfort him. But I don't think it helped. In the end, he didn't recognize us. Our whole family stood around his bed, but Danny couldn't have died more alone.

"I miss Danny now. I think about my brother every day. I can't help but wonder if what happened to Danny is going to happen to me too. When you have the AIDS virus, you always feel like a detective. Whenever I catch a cold, I get scared. For me, it's no longer just a matter of a runny nose or stuffed sinuses. I keep asking myself, 'Is this the start of it? Is my immune system on the blink? Am I going to get over this cold or is it my turn now?'

"I've tried to prepare myself for the most common physical symptoms of AIDS. But I don't think I could handle what happened to Danny. For me, the worst thing would be for my mind to go.

"I couldn't handle not being able to understand what's happening around me. It would be like dying before you actually stop breathing. I don't want to live out the last days of my life terrified the way Danny was. When that happens, the disease kills you in the worst possible way. It stops you from spending what little time you have left with your family.

"Right now, I still feel pretty good. I'm happy about that. Seeing what happened to Danny and having the virus myself has really changed the way I look at things. I've had a chance to work with a counselor and that helped too.

"I've learned to take one day at a time. I act differently now. I don't fight over little things anymore. I'm not going to let a silly disagreement spoil what could be a good day. Because when you have AIDS, you don't know how many good days are left."

Facts about AIDS

*What is considered safe behavior
during the AIDS epidemic?*

• Do not use IV drugs.[1]

• Sexually active individuals should have one mutually faithful uninfected partner. It is important to be aware of your partner's sexual history. With the spread of AIDS, it may be wise to wait until marriage to become sexually active.

• Do not engage in anal intercourse even with a condom.[2]

• Never assume that a person who looks and feels well is virus-free. Only a test for the AIDS antibody can ensure that.[3]

• Follow a sensible diet, get plenty of rest, and avoid recreational drugs. Such substances tend to damage a healthy immune system, making it more difficult to ward off bacteria and viruses.

• Be aware of new information about AIDS. As AIDS research continues, important developments will unfold. The more you know, the safer you'll remain.

Source Notes

KAREN

1. *AIDS: The Social Impact* (pamphlet), Weymouth, Massachusetts: Life Skills Education, Inc., 1988, 1.

ALLEN

1. Roland James. *Understanding AIDS*. Irvine, California: Century House Publications, Inc., 1988, 21.

JACKIE

1. "AIDS: What we know" (complete medical report), *McCall's*, April 1987, 144.

ALLISON

1. "Understanding AIDS: A Message From the Surgeon General," Rockville, Maryland: U.S. Department of Health and Human Services, 1988, 3.

MARIA

1. Ibid., p. 6.
2. "AIDS: What we know" (complete medical report), *McCall's*,
   April 1987, 145.

PAUL

1. "Understanding AIDS: A Message From the Surgeon General," 3.
2. Ibid.
3. Ibid., p. 5.

For More Information

Further information regarding AIDS may be obtained by contacting the following organizations:

AZT Hotline at the National Institutes of Health: (800) 843–9388; 8 A.M. to midnight (EST), seven days a week
Centers for Disease Control AIDS Hotline: (800) 342–AIDS; twenty-four hours a day, seven days a week
National Cancer Institute AIDS Information Hotline: (800) 4–CANCER; 9 A.M. to 4:30 P.M. (all time zones), Monday through Friday
National Gay Task Force AIDS Information Hotline (800) 221–7044; 3 P.M. to 9 P.M. (EST), Monday through Friday. (212) 529–1604 in New York
National Sexually Transmitted Diseases Hotline: (800) 227–8922; 8 A.M. to 8 P.M. (PST), Monday through Friday.

INFORMATIONAL GROUPS

American Association of Physicians for Human Rights, P.O. Box 14366, San Francisco, CA 94114; (415) 558–9353

American Red Cross AIDS Education Program, 17th and D Street, N.W., Washington, DC 20006; (202) 639–3223 or contact your local Red Cross chapter

Gay Men's Health Crisis, P.O. Box 274, 132 West 24th Street, New York, NY 10011; (212) 807–7035

Hispanic AIDS Forum c/o PRACA, 853 Broadway, Suite 2007, New York, NY 10003; (212) 870–1864

Los Angeles AIDS Project, 1362 Santa Monica Boulevard, Los Angeles, CA 90046; (213) 876–AIDS

Minority Task Force on AIDS, Director, Suki Ports, 92nd Street and Nicholas Avenue, Apt. 1B, New York, NY 10026

Mothers of AIDS Patients, c/o Barbara Peabody, 3043 E Street, San Diego, CA 92102; (619) 234–3432

AIDS Project Los Angeles, 3670 Wilshire Boulevard, Suite 300, Los Angeles, CA 90010; (213) 876–AIDS

San Francisco AIDS Foundation, 333 Valencia Street, 4th floor, San Francisco, CA 94103; (415) 863–2437

To receive a copy of the Surgeon General's report on AIDS free of charge, write to AIDS, Box 14252, Washington, DC 20044, or call (202) 245–6867.

For Further Reading

If you are interested in learning more about AIDS, the following books and articles may be helpful.

BOOKS

Hyde, Margaret O., and Forsyth, Elizabeth. *Know About AIDS*. New York: Walker, 1987.

Landau, Elaine. *Sexually Transmitted Diseases*. Hillside, New Jersey: Enslow, 1986.

Langone, John. *AIDS: The Facts*. Boston: Little Brown, 1988.

Levert, Susan. *AIDS: In Search of a Killer*. New York: Julian Messner, 1987.

Norse, Alan E. *AIDS*. New York: Franklin Watts, 1986.

Silverstein, Alvin, and Silverstein, Virginia B. *AIDS: Deadly Threat*. Hillside, New Jersey: Enslow, 1986.

ARTICLES

"AIDS Again" (future prevention) (column) by Robert Bazell. *New Republic* 199 (July 18, 1988), p. 15.

"AIDS: a Bad Way to Die—a Prison Epidemic," il. *Newsweek* 109 (March 23, 1987), p. 30.

"AIDS and Civil Rights" by Glen Allen. *Maclean's* 101 (Oct. 3, 1988), p. 50.

"AIDS and Home Buyers" by William Giese. *Changing Times* 42 (Oct. 1988), p. 18.

"AIDS Epidemiology: Women and Drugs" by Sarah Boxer, il. *Discover* 8 (July 1987), p. 12.

"AIDS: How Wide the Cover-up?" (Liberace's death), il. *U.S. News & World Report* 102 (Feb. 23, 1987), p. 8.

"AIDS in the Workplace: a New Ruling Restricts Protection for Victims" by Matt Clark, il. *Newsweek* 108 (July 7, 1986), p. 82.

"AIDS: Prejudice and Progress; of an Eighth-grader, a Football-player, and Infected Flies" (Ryan White) by Joe Levine, il. *Time* 128 (Sept 8, 1986), p. 68.

"AIDS Report Draws Tepid Response" by William Booth. *Science* 241 (Aug. 12, 1988), p. 778.

"AIDS: Safe Sex" by Lindsay Van Gelder, il. *Ms.* 15 (April 1987), p. 64.

"AIDS: Taking Action." *National Review* 40 (July 8, 1988), p. 17.

"AIDS: What We Know Now" (Complete Medical Report) by David R. Zimmerman and Kenneth K. Goldstein. *McCall's* 114 (April 1987), p. 143.

"And How Do Men Feel Now About Monogamy" (Sex From Now On) by Peter Mehiman, il. *Glamour* 86 (July 1988), p. 157.

"Artist Niki de Saint Phalle Sketches Lifesaving Truths for teen-agers unwary of AIDS" by Susan Reed, il. *People Weekly* 29 (Jan. 11, 1988), p. 51.

"The Charge: AIDS Assault; Is the Virus a Weapon?" (charging AIDS carriers with using the disease as a weapon) by Eric Press, il. *Newsweek* 109 (June 22, 1987), p. 25.

"Dangerous Leaks in the AIDS' Lab." *Discover* 8 (Dec. 1987), p. 14.

"Discrimination on Trial: HIV carriers have rights too" by Mark Gevisser, il. *The Nation* 248 (May 21, 1988), p. 710.

"A Doctor Can Easily Skirt the AIDS Issue by Attributing an AIDS Death to a Malignancy or Pneumonia, Two of the Common Conditions that Can Often Bring on an AIDS-related Death" by Robert C. Gallo. *Omni* 10 (Dec. 1987), p. 10.

"Ebony Interview with U.S. Surgeon General C. Everett Koop, M.D." by Laura B. Randolph, il. *Ebony* 43 (Sept. 1988), p. 154.

"Fear of Death and Disease" (AIDS) by Ann Finlavson and Mark Leiren-Young, il. *McLean's* 100 (Jan. 12, 1987), p. 32.

"The Fears and Facts of Sex Now" by Rosemary Ellis, il. *Glamour* 86 (July 1988), p. 154.

"Fighting AIDS Discrimination: New Laws and Court Decisions Help Those Singled Out by Tests" by Alain L. Sanders, il. *Time* 132 (Sept. 5, 1988), p. 38.

"For Better or Worse. This Is the Story of a Husband, a Wife and a Moment of Indiscretion. This Is a Story of AIDS" by Kathryn Casey, il. *Ladies Home Journal* 104 (May 1987), p. 89.

"His Love for a Brother with AIDS Brings Morton Downey's Compassion Out of the Closet" by Jack Friedman, il. *People Weekly* 29 (June 20, 1988), p. 44.

"House Approves AIDS Bill by Overwhelming Margin" by Irvin Molotsky, il. *The New York Times* 138 (Sept. 24, 1988), p. 6 (N), col. 1.

"How AIDS Affects Us All" by Diane Salvatore and Sharon Aborn, il. *Ladies Home Journal* 104 (Oct. 1987), p. 119.

"How to Ask about Sex and Get Honest Answers" by Gina Kolata, il. *Science* (April 24, 1987), p. 387.

"I'm Dying—AIDS Is Your Problem Now" (includes author's observations before dying from AIDS) (One Year in the Epidemic) by James Hurley, il. *Newsweek* 110 (Aug. 10, 1987), p. 38.

"Inescapable Problem: AIDS in Prison" by Marsha F. Goldsmith. *JAMA (The Journal of the American Medical Association)* 268 (Dec. 11, 1987), p. 3215.

"Inside the Illegal AIDS Drug Trade" (mixing greed and good) (dextran sulfate) by Joshua Hammer, il. *Newsweek* 112 (Aug. 15, 1988), p. 41.

"Judge Bars Release of AIDS Test" by Dennis Hevesi. *The New York Times* 138 (Oct. 20, 1988), p. 9 (N), col. 1.

"Kansas Judge Bars Doctor's Release of Positive for AIDS Virus" (American Civil Liberties Union Case) by Dennis Hevesi. *The New York Times* 138 (Oct. 9, 1988), p. A16 (L), col. 3.

"Last Call" (AIDS policy) (column) by Fred Barnes. *New Republic* 199 (Oct. 10, 1988), p. 10.

"A Lawsuit over Rock's Estate Exposes Scandal—and Asserts a Lover's Right to Know" (Rock Hudson) by Scott Haller, il. *People Weekly* 24 (Nov. 25, 1985), p. 52.

"Legal Rights and Duties in the AIDS Epidemic" by Bernard M. Dickens. *Science* 239 (Feb. 5, 1988).

"Legal-service Group Files Suit Against Segregating Inmates with AIDS" (New York) by Elizabeth Kolbert. *The New York Times* 130 (Sept. 28, 1988), p. 82 (L), col. 2.

"The Long Agony of Shirley Fish" (family members are AIDS victims) by Georgette Bennell, il. *McCall's* 114 (April 1987), p. 148.

"A Man's Report on His Dwindling Options" by Bruce Weber, il. *Glamour* 86 (July 1988), p. 152.

"A New Clue in the AIDS Mystery: Evidence That the Disease Was Here in the '60's" by Matt Clark and Daniel Shapiro, il. *Newsweek* 110 (Nov. 9, 1987), p. 62.

"No Legacy" (White House Watch—AIDS policy) (column) by Fred Barnes. *New Republic* 198 (July 4, 1988), p. 11.

"$1 Million Award in AIDS Suit" (brother barred from school because of exposure to AIDS virus). *The New York Times* 138 (Sept. 30, 1988), p. 85 (L), col. 5.

"The Politicization of AIDS" by D. Keith Mano. *National Review* 38 (Feb. 28, 1986), p. 59.

"Private Passions & Public health: For Some People It Takes More Than an AIDS Test to Temper Fatal Attractions" (includes two related articles) by Kevin Krajick, il. *Psychology Today* 22 (May 1988), p. 50.

"Right to Bar Treatment by Any with AIDS Virus Weighted." *The New York Times* 137 (Sept. 16, 1988), p. B7 (L), col. 2.

"Ruling on AIDS Test for Rape Suspect Divides Experts" (accused rapist not required to submit to AIDS test) by Dennis Hevesi. *The New York Times* 138 (Oct. 16, 1988), p. 12 (N), col. 3.

"Should HIV Carriers Have Secrets?", il. *Time* 132 (Nov. 7, 1988), p. 36.

"Stockholm Speakers on Adolescents and AIDS: Catch Them Before They Catch It" (Fourth International Conference on AIDS) by Marsha F. Goldsmith. *JAMA* (*The Journal of the American Medical Association*) 260 (Aug. 12, 1988), p. 757.

"Straight Talk" (heterosexuals and AIDS) by John Tiernay, il. *Rolling Stone* (Nov. 17, 1988), p. 122.

"Tracking the Spread of AIDS" by Nora Underwood. *McLean's* 100 (Aug. 31, 1987), p. 32.

"The Untouchables: in a New York STD Clinic Dedicated Doctors Struggle with Despair and Dodging the Odds" (AIDS clinic case study) by Paul Perry. *American Health: Fitness of Body and Mind* 7 (June 1988), p. 56.

"What Can We Believe? For heterosexuals It's the Doubts, not the Data That Terrifies" (AIDS disease) by Judy Ismach. *American Health: Fitness of Body and Mind* 7 (June 1988), p. 53.

"A Woman with AIDS: One Year Later" by Lisa DePaulo, il. *Philadelphia Magazine* 79 (May 1988), p. 114.

INDEX

About the Author

Elaine Landau received her BA degree from New York University in English and Journalism and a master's in Library and Information Science from Pratt Institute.

Ms. Landau has worked as a newspaper reporter, an editor, and a youth services librarian, but she believes that many of her most fascinating as well as rewarding hours have been spent researching and writing books and articles on contemporary issues for young people.

Ms. Landau makes her home in Sparta, New Jersey.